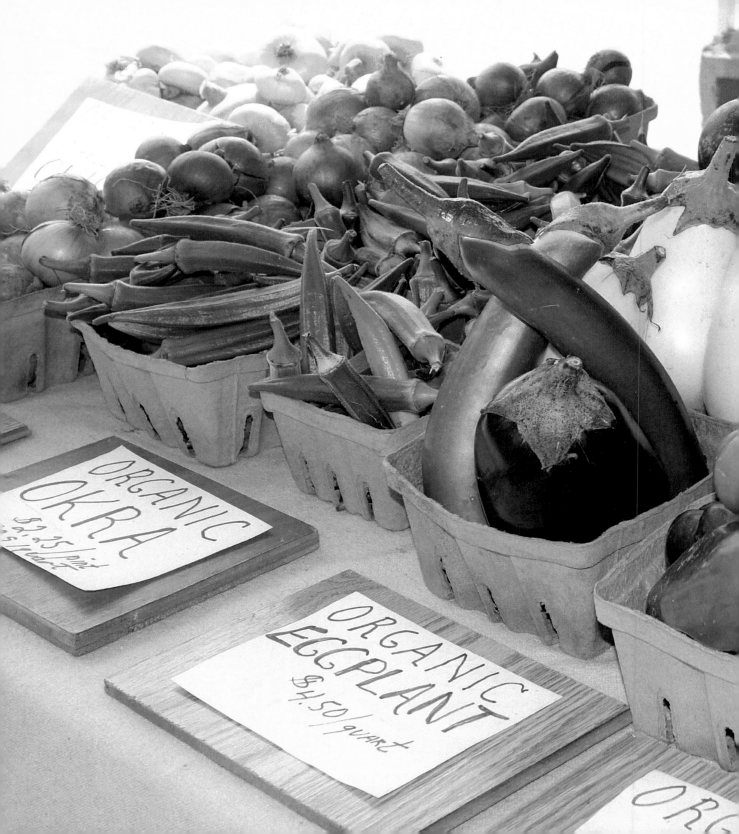

Eat with the Seasons

Simple Recipes to Inspire Health, Wellness & Weight Control

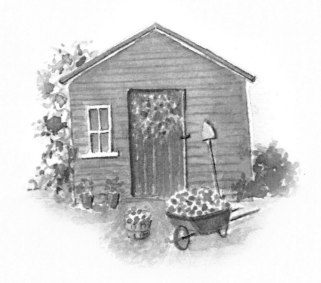

Michelle C. Wohlfarth

Second Edition May 2013
Second Printing 2014
© 2013 Michelle C. Wohlfarth
℗ 2013 Healthy Living Kitchen, LLC

Library of Congress Cataloguing in-Publication Data is available upon request.

Additional art direction, design & layout by Sherri L. Long
of Double Click Design, www.dcdpublications.com

Cover art by watercolor artist, Linda J. Berry, from Linda Berry Patch
You can see more of her work at www.lindaberrypatch.com

Visit us on the web:
www.healthylivingkitchenpa.com

PRINTED IN THE U.S.A.

TABLE OF CONTENTS

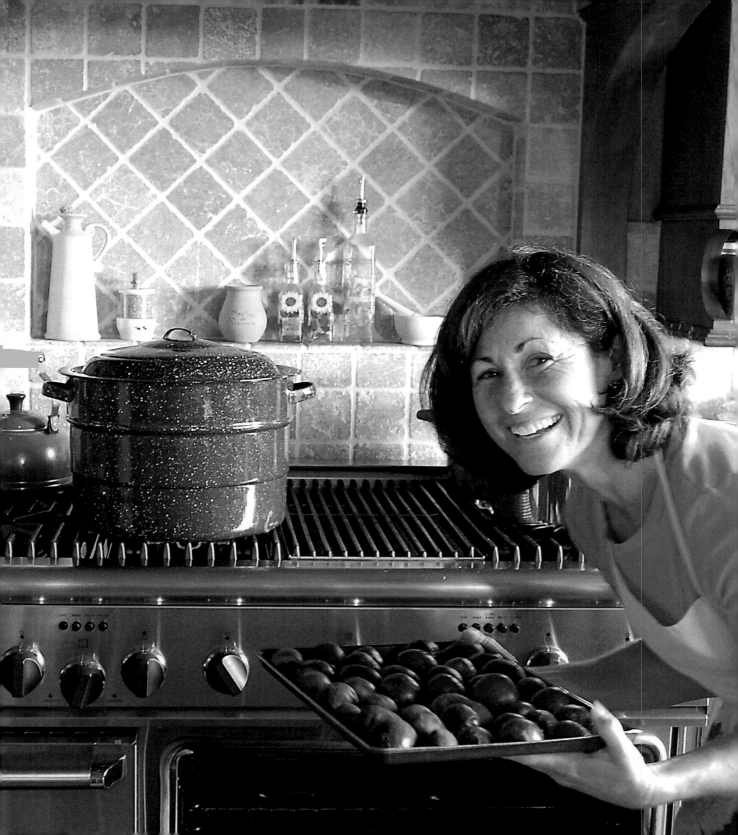

ACKNOWLEDGEMENTS

Needless to say, this book has been a journey for me. The recipes come from all aspects of my life. Whether from my childhood, my travels, my cooking experience, or my education, eating and cooking delicious food has always been a part of me. I first want to thank my husband, Donnie for being the best recipe tester there is....he loves everything I make!!! His loving encouragement has made my cooking experience an easy road to travel. He continues to inspire me to follow my dream. I thank my French mother, Jacqueline for being the catalyst for eating healthy whole foods. Little did I know when I was young, the incredible education I was getting every night at dinner. She managed to make a gourmet meal out of eggs just by using herbs and garlic. I remember wishing we had soda, ring dings and frozen dinners in our cupboards like other "normal" people. Thanks Mom for not knowing! Although I sometimes ate those foods, it was a habit I never had to break! We were lucky enough to have French relatives and go to France very often. I learned an appreciation for the simplicity of wholesome products coming right from the local producers. It tastes so much better when someone's heart and soul is in the growing and making. I thank my children who are the best eaters ever! They have such open minds and will try just about anything. Granted we had our crash and burn meals (like the chickpea soup that they will never let me forget), but they were patient with all my new experiments as well as my herbal medicine cures that tasted terrible. Dinner was always a time to be together and share our stories. It continues to be a time of celebration for our family. I thank my sister Cathy who has always been an advisor and cheerleader for the things I do. She is my honest critic who will always tell me the truth for the good of my purpose and is a true supporter. Thank you to my colleague Beth Pasqualina who has helped me work through many of the programs HLK has offered, as well as serving as my own private health coach. And last, but not least, I want to thank all the people along the way who have contributed to my continuing growth at Healthy Kitchen. They supported my cooking classes and health sessions and spread the word. So to my mother-in-law Marianne, Brenda HF, Kim S., Jackie O., Liz M., Andrea L., and all of the other wonderful people I have met in my classes I say thank you so much for your heartfelt support.

Keep It Simple!

(The reason for writing this book.)

Eating with the seasons is a framework for living that goes back to basics and helps simplify all the jargon about what's healthy and what's not. It's about eating a whole foods diet that helps bring joy back into eating, cooking and living in a way that no "diet" can. It releases the grip of "shoulds" and "should nots" and helps us move into our body's language.

My hope is that when you follow this book for one year, it will help bring enthusiasm and joy into your daily routine of living; that it can help you re-balance your body, your metabolism and your life, if necessary. In an effort to help simplify all the confusion about clean eating and balanced living, I have found that living in tune with the natural rhythms of the seasons is a compass that guides me. When I'm feeling a little off kilter I tune in to what's going on seasonally, eat seasonal foods, observe what's growing, exercise outside, or just sit outside for a time. This is very grounding and therapeutic and helps to keep me in tune to my body and soul. Staying in touch with the seasons helps me to find my soul expression. I delight in the subtle changes of light and color, the flowers and trees that offer so much variation, and the changes in weather. The cold windy weather of winter always makes the thought of a hot sticky summer that much nicer.

My hope is that this book will help others find their rhythm in the "influences" of each season, no matter how subtle they may be. Take a little time each day to notice what is happening all around you, and what is happening right inside you. Where are you shifting and what is your body trying to tell you? Enjoy every moment of your new discoveries.

Bon Appétit!

Michelle

Author:
MICHELLE C. WOHLFARTH

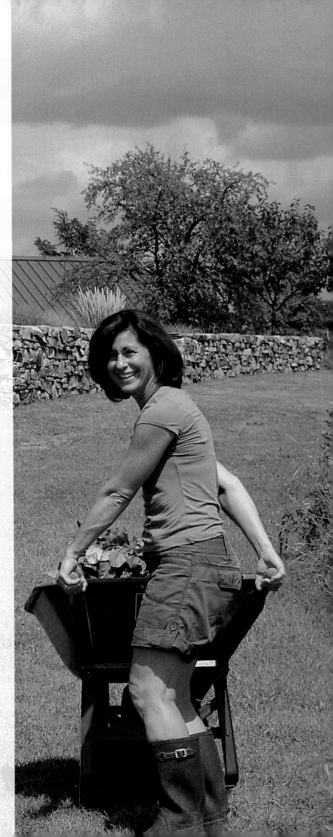

Founder of The Healthy Living Kitchen, Michelle is a Holistic Health Educator and Certified Nutrition Coach. She created The Healthy Living Kitchen in 2005 to follow her passion for cooking wholesome food, caring for the earth, and keeping all things in their natural order. Her mantra is, "eating healthy is easy", and her mission is to live joyfully and to assist others in achieving the life they desire, one small step at a time.

She earned Certification in Food Therapy in 2011 from The Natural Gourmet Institute for Health and Culinary Arts in New York City, where she studied under the Institute's founder, Annemarie Colbin, Ph.D. Her certification complements credentials as a Holistic Health Coach from the Institute for Integrative Nutrition in New York in 2004, and her completion of the Master Chef Series under Chef Peter Berley, at the Natural Gourmet Institute in 2009. Her objective is to use food therapies in a way that supports a whole health practice and offers clients practical ways to make changes that favor health and well-being. The study of Plant Science and French as an undergraduate at The University of New Hampshire led her on the path to study culinary and medicinal herbs. After 15 years of practicing on her family, she pursued a Certificate in Herbal Studies in 2003 from Mt. Nittany Institute in State College, PA. She continues to apply her knowledge of herbs in cooking, and in healing the body, mind, and spirit, as well as integrating her knowledge of healing with whole foods.

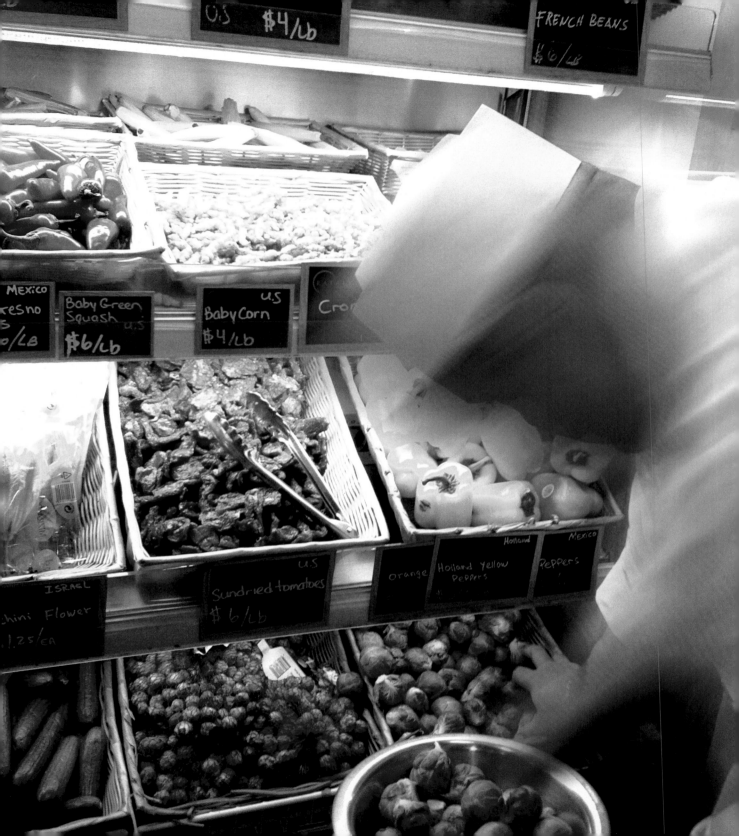

How to Begin

"In the beginner's mind there are many possibilities,
but in the expert's mind there are few."
— SHUNRYU SUZUKI

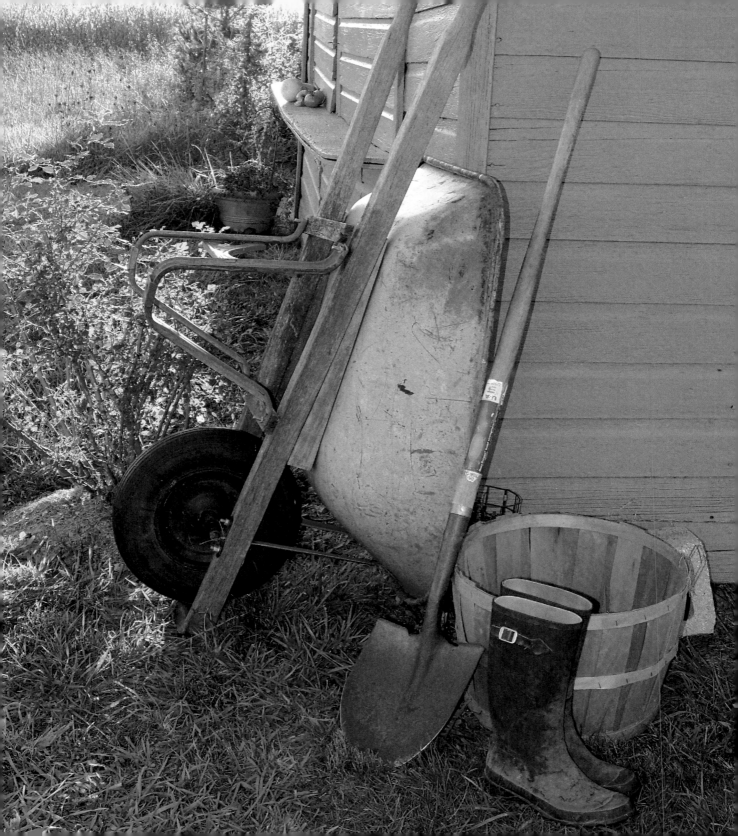

How To Use This Book

I have set the framework of this book for use on many levels depending on where you are now. My suggestion is to open to the season we are in at the moment and begin cooking. From there you can determine where you want to go.

Here are 3 suggestions;

1. Use the book for new recipe ideas by beginning to use the menus and recipes as you follow the seasons and stay in tune with your body.

   In the process of making the recipes CLEAN OUT YOUR PANTRY of old, unused products and spices. Discard. This has a very cleansing effect. Begin to stock your pantry with the new wholesome ingredients called for in these recipes. That does not mean you run out and buy all new ingredients. That would be too costly! As you finish up one of your old ingredients, like white refined flour, purchase a new more wholesome product, like spelt, to replace it. This way you will restock your pantry in a more economical way.

2. For the person wishing to learn more, read the 'How to Begin' chapter for tips on new ingredients, information on food and health, how to stock your pantry and refrigerator, what's in season, easy solution ideas, and some basic recipes to get you started.

3. For a little more in-depth use, and to help you achieve more joy and balance in your life, do the above, but also complete the 'Seasonal Plan' and 'Circle of Life' for each season. Set a date with yourself each season to do the exercises. I like to do them at the beginning of each season on the spring/fall equinox and summer/winter solstice. This sets me up for a year of energetic balance.

Enjoy and please share your stories with me on my blog at http://joyfulljourney.com.

What's In Season?

Farmer's markets are a fun, community place to go. Supporting your local market helps our farmers earn a living providing us with wholesome food. The more we buy from our local farmers, the more diversified and sustainable our food system will be. Shopping at "producer only" markets makes the foods in season clear, and prices are usually more reasonable from your local farmer.

The more you can support your local farmer, the more farmers will be able to earn a living producing wholesome food for us to eat. If it's difficult to get to a market then consider joining a CSA (community supported agriculture) where you buy into a share at the beginning of the season and then pick it up weekly at a nearby "drop-off" location. Or, try a Virtual Farmers Market like ours, where you order online from your farmer and pick up your order at a nearby drop-off location.

There are so many reasons to shop locally. Shopping locally;

- tastes better
- is fun and easy
- supports the local economy and helps it grow
- reduces our energy footprint, which in turns helps to reduce pollution and damage to the environment
- builds community support
- keeps us healthy and vibrant

SUPPORT YOUR LOCAL FARMER!

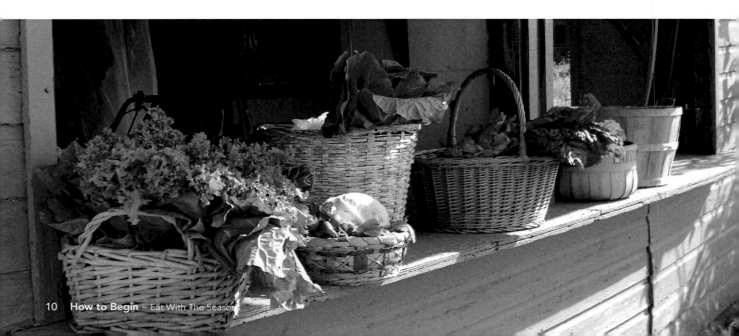

SPRING
Spring Vegetables
- Asparagus
- Scallions
- Mushrooms
- Leeks
- Peas
- Artichokes
- Lettuce, spring greens mix
- Arugula
- Spinach
- New Potatoes
- Radishes
- Wild Greens, like dandelion greens
- Watercress
- Sprouts

Spring Fruit
- Avocado
- Rhubarb
- Strawberries

SUMMER
Summer Herbs
- Basil
- Cilantro
- Parsley
- Dill
- Other Herbs like thyme, rosemary, tarragon, oregano, marjoram, lavender

Summer Vegetables
- Corn
- Cucumbers
- Eggplant
- Fennel
- Green Beans
- Kohlrabi
- Okra
- Peppers
- Tomatoes
- Summer Squash
- Zucchini

Summer Fruit
- Apricots
- Berries
- Cherries
- Melon
- Nectarines
- Peaches
- Plums

FALL
Fall Vegetables
- Beets
- Broccoli
- Kale
- Brussels Sprouts
- Cauliflower
- Collards
- Swiss Chard
- Pumpkin
- Winter Squashes, like hubbard, acorn, butternut

Fall Fruit
- Grapes
- Apples
- Pears
- Cranberries

WINTER
Winter vegetables
- Beets
- Cabbage
- Chilies
- Carrots
- Parsnips
- Potatoes
- Rutabagas
- Sweet Potatoes
- Turnips

Winter Fruit
- Pomegranate
- Citrus
- Persimmons
- Dried Fruit

Spring/Winter Grains
- Amaranth
- Buckwheat
- Millet
- Oats
- Quinoa
- Brown Rice
- Rye
- Wheat

Summer/Fall Grains
- Barley
- Rice
- Some Rye
- Some Oats
- Some Wheat

HERE ARE SUGGESTIONS FOR A DILEMMA PROOF PANTRY.
TAILOR YOUR PANTRY TO YOUR NEEDS...

CANNED OR JARRED GOODS
- Beans like Chickpeas, Cannellini, Kidney, Great Northern, Chili Beans
- Tomatoes, diced, whole and crushed
- Tomato Sauce
- Tomato Paste
- Canned Fish, Tuna and Salmon, Sardines
- Artichoke Hearts
- Sun Dried Tomatoes
- Anchovies
- Roasted Red Peppers
- Nut Butters like Almond, Peanut Butter, Tahini
- Canned Pumpkin
- Applesauce with no sugar added
- Brown Rice Sweetener
- Pure Maple Syrup
- Raw Local Honey

OILS
- Extra Virgin Olive Oil - first cold pressed (unrefined is best)
- Coconut Oil - extra virgin
- Sesame Oil

VINEGARS
- Balsamic Vinegar
- Red Wine Vinegar
- Brown Rice Vinegar

CONDIMENTS
- Apple Cider Vinegar - Umeboshi Plum Vinegar
- Dijon Mustard
- Tamari soy sauce, refrigerate after opening
- Sesame Seed Blend and sea salt combinations
- Sea vegetables (kombu, wakame)

DRY GOODS
- Healthy Granola without any added sweeteners
- Muesli
- Whole Grain Flours like spelt, whole wheat, oat, corn, garbanzo

WHOLE GRAINS
- Quinoa, Steel-Cut Oats, Brown Rice, Brown Basmati Rice, Bulgur Wheat, Barley, Millet, Whole Grain Pasta, Udon and Soba Noodles

BOXED, LOW-SODIUM VEGETABLE AND/OR CHICKEN BROTH

WHOLE WHEAT PANKO BREADCRUMBS

NUTS & SEEDS (pick your favorites and remember they easily go rancid)
- Almonds, Cacao Nibs, Walnuts, Pine Nuts, Pumpkin Seeds, Sesame Seeds, Sunflower Seeds

BEANS AND LEGUMES
- Chickpeas, Lentils, Split Peas, Black Beans

DRIED FRUIT
- Apricots, Dates, Prunes, Raisins

HERBS & SPICES
- Black Peppercorns, Chili Powder, Cinnamon, Crushed Red Pepper, Cumin, Garlic Powder, Ginger, Herb Blends like Herbes de Provence or Italian Blend, Onion Powder, Oregano, Rosemary, Sage, Thyme
- Sea Salt and/or Kosher Salt

OTHER
- Onions, Garlic, Potatoes, Sweet Potatoes

DILEMMA PROOF REFRIGERATOR

This list can be helpful for stocking your fridge with clean food that will enable you to whip up a healthy meal anytime.

DAIRY
- Carton of eggs, (free range, organic preferred)
- Low fat milk or full fat if preferred, organic
- Plain yogurt (full fat preferred)
- Greek yogurt
- Plain kefir
- Variety of cheeses like Parmesan, Feta, Goat, Swiss
- Cottage cheese

TOFU/TEMPEH/MISO

ASSORTED VEGETABLES
Go with things that are in season but keep the following on hand always;
- Carrots
- Celery
- Leafy greens like kale, Swiss chard, spinach, collards
- Onions
- Garlic
- Mixed greens or lettuce
- Avocados
- Leeks

ASSORTED FROZEN VEGETABLES
- Spinach
- Broccoli
- Kale
- Corn (NON GMO)
- Peas
- Mixed, and other family favorites

ASSORTED FRESH FRUIT
Best to keep seasonal fruit on hand
- Apples
- Lemons and limes

ASSORTED FROZEN FRUIT
- Berries like blueberries and strawberries
- Mangoes
- Bananas

CONDIMENTS
- Salsa
- Dijon style mustard
- Clean Mayonnaise without additives
- Tamari Soy Sauce
- Horseradish
- Miso
- Hummus
- Nut Butters like Peanut butter and Almond butter
- Spreads like all fruit jams
- Pure maple syrup
- Wheat Germ and/or Flaxseeds

OTHER FROZEN ITEMS
- Frozen fish like wild caught Alaskan salmon or other favorites
- Frozen chicken or turkey cutlets
- Frozen whole chicken
- Ground turkey
- Ground grass-fed beef or bison
- Pre-made salmon burgers or veggie burgers
- Homemade veggie and/or chicken broth

ALTERNATIVE MILKS
- Almond
- Rice
- Coconut

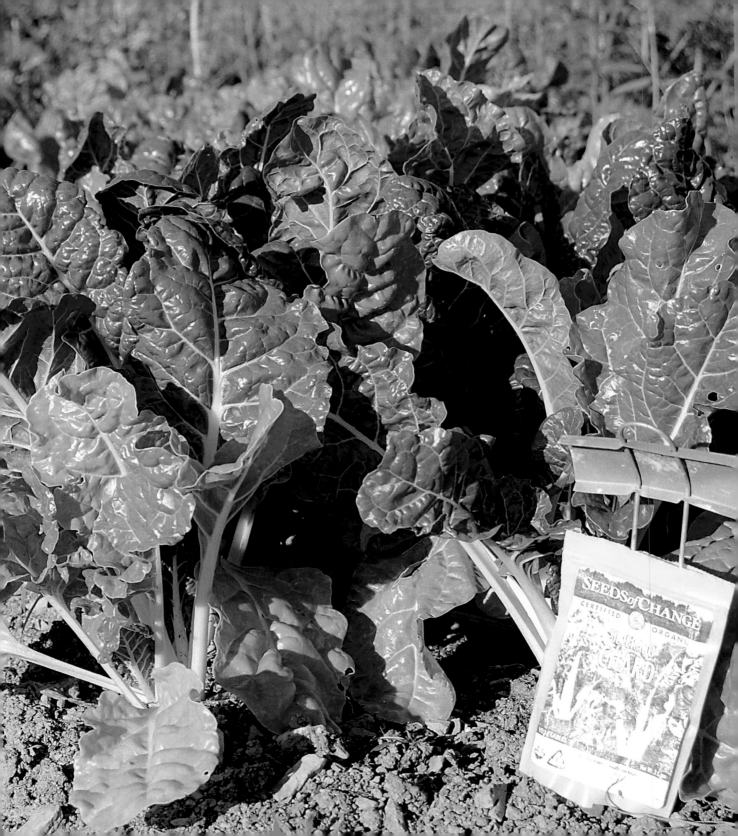

Start With The Basics

The Importance Of Chewing

Eating begins with the simple art of chewing. Chewing leads to smooth digestion and greater assimilation of nutrients because it initiates the release of digestive enzymes, which begin to break down food. I was always a slow eater just because it was in my nature. I only realized the value of my "skill" when I began studying nutrition and the digestive system. I have noticed that I chew less when I am under stress or in a rush and this affects how I feel after my meal, as well as the flavor of my food.

Carbohydrate digestion begins in the mouth. Chewing turns grains and other complex carbohydrates into satisfying sugars and makes oils, proteins and minerals available for maximum absorption. Whole foods, especially whole grains, must be mixed with saliva and chewed until liquid to release their full nutritional value. In addition, the more whole carbohydrate foods are chewed, the sweeter they become. Because digestion becomes so efficient when you chew your food, your body will begin to feel wonderfully light.

How to chew properly:

- To get started in the habit of chewing correctly, try counting the chewing of each bite 30 to 50 times at the beginning of each meal. It helps to put down your fork between bites.

- Chew every mouthful of food at least 30 times each, until the food becomes liquid.

- Chewing breaks down food and makes it easier for the stomach and small intestine to digest.

- Saliva assists in the digestion of carbohydrates.

- Saliva also makes the food more alkaline, which creates less gas. (Gas is experienced in the stomach and intestine but can be caused by spleen imbalances.)

- If under pressure at meals, simply chew, and let the chewing relax you. Then you can enjoy the whole spectrum of tastes and aromas that make up the meal. Try to always chew for the allotted time you have to eat your meal. Whatever is left over at the end, save for later.

- Mindful chewing can be very relaxing and meditative. As you learn to chew your food you will probably find that you are enjoying the moment, the day, your life, much more.

WATER: ARE YOU DRINKING ENOUGH?

Water is the fluid of life. It's the most abundant nutrient in the body. It is essential for so many bodily functions including: blood circulation which carries heat and nourishment through the body, lymphatic system which processes and eliminates wastes and provides the ability to fight infections, the flow of urine, saliva, perspiration, tears, and sexual fluids, to name a few. (Elson Haas).

According to Paul Pitchford, water requirements are lessened by:

- a sedentary lifestyle
- the consumption of fruit, vegetables, and sprouted foods
- cold or damp climates

Water requirements are increased by:

- physical activity
- consumption of more meat, eggs, or salty foods
- fever condition
- dry, hot, or windy climates

How much water do we really need? Let your body do the talking.

Beans & Protein

What is protein? Protein is a component of food, called amino acids, that comes in many different forms. Amino Acids are the building blocks for major parts of a lean human body. They are crucial to the minute-by-minute regulation and maintenance of bodies. Therefore, your body makes its own supply of amino acids, and also must get some from food. Why is it important? Protein is a basic building block of cells and tissues needed to keep us strong. It is crucial for vital functions, regulation, and maintenance of our bodies. **Too little protein** can cause many problems; Common symptoms include: sugar and sweet cravings, feeling spacey and jittery, fatigue, weight loss, loss of healthy color on facial area, weak feeling, anemia, change in hair color and texture, skin inflammation (in severe cases), pot belly (in severe cases). **Too much** can also cause problems; Common symptoms include: low energy, constipation, dehydration, lethargic, heavy feeling, weight gain, sweet cravings, feeling "tight" or stiff joints, body becomes overly acidic, kidney function declines (due to the stress required to process excess proteins — kidney faces increased pressure to filter toxins and filter wastes), foul body odor, halitosis and calcium loss to compensate for acidic status in body.

So how do you know what to do? Protein has been a controversial subject in the U.S. Some people say we eat too much, others say we need more. There are diets that are mostly protein, then others that are high in carbohydrates. My belief is that we all need some protein in our daily diet. I love the 40-40-20 ratio (protein-complex carbohydrates-fat) as a good starting ground. It's important to take into consideration your heritage, blood type, activity level, weight, and how you feel when you eat protein. Not all proteins are equal and it's important to take note of how you feel after each. This is often the biggest indicator for you.

There are several sources of protein available; animal and vegetarian. Which source you choose is a personal choice. It's important to respect your body's needs, as well as the needs of the planet. **It is possible to eat meat and yet still abide by sustainable practices that are healthy for the earth and human consumption. Eating locally and humanely raised grass-fed beef, organically raised pork, wild, sustainably caught fish, pasture raised, organic poultry and eggs, and wild game is very important to the life of our planet. My philosophy is to eat less but eat high quality proteins.** When it comes to vegetarian sources it's important to eat high quality whole grains, fresh and dried beans, nuts and seeds, organically raised non-genetically modified soy products. Try reading the book by Michael Pollen called *The Omnivore's Dilemma* to find out more about the fundamental questions on what to eat and how our food sources affect our planet and our bodies or, catch the movie, *Food Inc.* to raise your awareness about what you are putting in your body. I think it's very important for all of us to have a connection to the food we eat and to take responsibility for the choices we make everyday. These other sources will help. I like to talk about beans as a source of protein because they are another wonderful and economic way to add high-quality, plant-based protein to your diet. They are high in iron, B vitamins and fiber, and are versatile enough that you may never tire of them. Many people struggle with digesting beans, which is why I have included the information on cooking. One of my "Basics" cooking classes is all about how to include this wonderful food in your diet. Beans stay fresh longer when stored in a cool, dark place (rather than on your countertop). Don't use beans that are more than a year old, as their nutrient content and digestibility are much lower. Also, old beans will not soften even with thorough cooking.

BASIC RECIPE TO COOK DRIED BEANS:

1. Check beans for rocks and broken beans, then wash.

2. Soak for 6 hours or overnight, using 4 cups of water per cup of beans. Small and medium-size beans may require less soaking – 4 hours. Note: If you've forgotten to presoak the beans, you can bring them to a boil in ample water to cover. Turn off the heat, cover the pot, and let stand for 1 hour.

3. Drain the beans and discard the soaking water. Always discard any loose skins before cooking, this decreases the chance of poor digestion.

4. Place the beans in a heavy pot and add 3 to 4 cups of fresh water (to cover).

5. Bring to a low boil and skim off the foam. Reduce to a simmer.

6. Add a small piece of kombu (seaweed), a few bay leaves or garlic cloves for flavor and better digestibility.

7. Cover, lower the temperature and simmer for the suggested time. Check beans 30 minutes before the minimum cooking time. Beans are done when the middle is soft.

8. About 10 minutes before the end of cooking time, add 1 teaspoon of unrefined sea salt.

9. Cook until beans are tender. Remove seaweed. You can use the beans with the broth for a soup or stew, or strain the liquid and use the beans in your recipe and retain the broth for a soup.

1 CUP DRY BEANS + COOKING TIME

adzuki	1 to 1½ hrs	lentils - red*	20 to 30 mins
anasazi	1½ to 2 hrs	lima beans	1 hr
black (turtle)	1½ to 2 hrs	split peas*	45 mins
black-eyed peas	30 to 45 mins	pinto*	1½ to 2 hrs
cannellini	1 to 1½ hrs	navy	1½ to 2 hrs
chickpeas (garbanzos)	1½ to 2 hrs	mung	1 hr
cranberry	1½ to 2 hrs	red kidney	2 to 3 hrs
great northern	1 to 1½ hrs	yellow or black soybeans	4 to 6 hrs
lentils - brown & french	30 to 45 mins		

Does not require soaking

Digestibility — some people have difficulty digesting beans and other legumes and develop gas, intestinal problems, irritability, and unclear thinking. Here are a few techniques for preparing and eating legumes that alleviate most problems.

- Chew beans thoroughly and realize that even small amounts have high nutritional and healing value. Experiment with your level of digestibility. Adzuki beans, lentils, mung beans, and peas digest more easily. Remember to cook the beans with kombu seaweed to help with digestibility.

- Avoid giving legumes to children under 18 months because they have not developed the gastric enzymes to digest them properly. Except in the case of an allergy, soybean products, fresh peas, and green beans are usually tolerated.

GLORIOUS GREENS

Leafy greens are one of the most lacking foods in the standard American diet. These gems are the first food I recommend to people to add to their meals, and the darker green the better. Just the color green reminds me of spring, energy, refreshing and renewal.

Nutritionally speaking, greens are high in calcium, magnesium, iron, potassium, phosphorus, zinc, and Vitamins A, C, E, and K. They are high in fiber and chlorophyll. Chlorophyll has been shown to stop the spread of bacteria, fungi, and micro-organisms (candida) and promote the growth of beneficial intestinal flora. These foods help lift mucus, clear congestion, and discharge toxins from the lungs. Greens are liver-supporting foods that help to rejuvenate and cleanse the liver, especially the cereal grasses like wheat grass and spirulina. They are blood purifiers, energizers, and cancer prevention foods because they are high in antioxidants. They are a great source of easily absorbable calcium and help to regulate calcium in the body. Most people get their greens from eating salads. I would like to introduce you to leafy greens beyond salad like, kale, collards, bok choy, and, I include broccoli and cabbage in this group. These are all very hardy and flexible vegetables. Swiss chard, beet greens, and spinach are all high in iron and other nutrients, but they do contain oxalic acid which has been shown to deplete calcium from your bones and teeth. It's best to eat these in moderation and with proteins that balance them out.

When you make salads try adding light cleansing greens like watercress, dandelion, escarole, arugula, endive, parsley, and wild greens. So many choices and each has its own flavor.

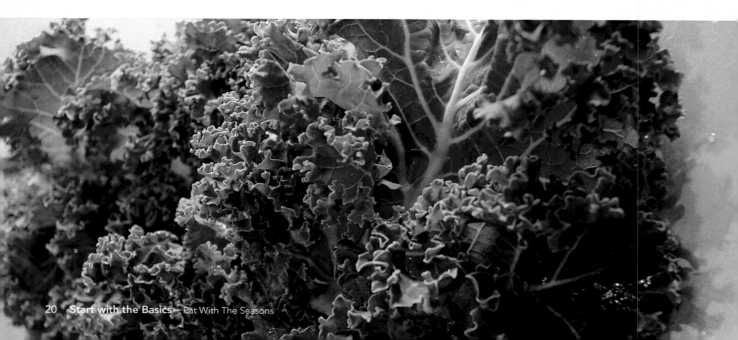

Kale is queen when it comes to phytonutrient content. Try some of the recipes in the book to decide how you can add about 3 to 5 servings of greens per day. Boiling some of the tougher, more bitter greens like collards and kale will take some of the bitter flavor out and still contain significant levels of calcium, iron, Vitamin A, and Vitamin C. Adding these to soups and stews and casseroles is so easy. Steaming greens will make them more fibrous and tight and can be excellent for those trying to lose weight. Raw salads have their place, especially in the warmer weather, but heating the greens can help make nutrients more available for the body to absorb, and helps eliminate any parasites that may be on the food. I will often buy big bunches of kale and wash and cut it up and put it in the refrigerator to pull out as needed. I add it to omelets, soups, casseroles and even eat it just plain. I can always tell when my body needs more green! It's important to buy these vegetables grown organically, as much as possible, so that you are not ingesting herbicides and pesticides along with all the important nutrients. Cook enough at one time to eat for several meals.

I would like to say a word about another green vegetable that I love; **sea vegetables... or seaweed**. You will often see recipes calling for kombu or wakame and these are both seaweeds that I love to use. There are many other seaweeds out there but I will focus on these for the time being. In general, sea vegetables contain the greatest amount and broadest range of minerals, vitamins, amino acids, calcium, and iron of any organism. Our blood contains all 100 or so minerals and trace elements found in the ocean water. Seaweeds contain these same minerals and elements in the most assimilable form of plant tissue. They also contain fiber, calcium and chlorophyll, are low in fat, and have many healing properties. They are used to lower cholesterol and blood pressure, regulate blood sugars, detoxify radioactive elements, heavy metals and free radicals. They can rejuvenate the lungs and GI tract, ease depression, stimulate production of immune cells, relieve menopausal symptoms, nourish the endocrine system, promote healthy thyroid function, help with weight loss, alkalize the blood, soften hardened masses in the body, as a diuretic, and to alleviate liver stagnancy, just to name a few! They are truly a wonder food!

Seaweeds provide B-complex vitamins, antioxidants, essential amino acids and fatty acids and a high source of calcium. Wakame has 10-times more calcium than milk. Kelp has 4-times more iron than beef, and triple the amount of iodine than shellfish and other fish. This is a great food to add to the diet. I usually cook my grains and beans with kombu to add nutrients and help with digestibility. I love to put seaweed sprinkles on my dishes for added flavor and nutrients. You can often find these in your local health food store or you may have to order. (See Resources on page 248 for sources). It's worth the effort to get used to working with these amazing sea vegetables.

GRAINS & BALANCE

Whole grains have been a central part of the human diet since the beginning of civilization when we went from being hunter-gatherers to settling down in agrarian communities. Whole grains contributed to building strong, lean bodies. Each country had its grains based on climate and availability. In the Americas we had corn. India and Asia had rice. Africa had sorghum and the Middle East had wheat. Scotland had oats and Russia had buckwheat. Europe had a mix of many, such as wheat, rice, millet. Nowadays we can find all of these fabulous grains in most grocery stores. Whole grains are a great source of nutritional support. They are high in fiber, an excellent source of B-Vitamins, which help calm the nervous system, high in iron, and they contain all the major nutrient groups needed by the body, as in complex carbohydrates, protein, fats, vitamins and minerals. They are very supportive to stress resistance, ensure steady blood sugar levels, build the body up, and have been shown to help with heart health. I find them to be very versatile in meal preparation. They keep very well in the refrigerator and busy people can prepare larger amounts and reheat later or use in multiple recipes. They have kept people fit and healthy through civilizations.

So if grains have been part of our diet for all these years why are people more overweight now? What has changed? We still eat wheat and corn and oats and other grains. The BIG difference is in the refining process. What we eat now are refined grains, not whole grains. When you eat most breads, bagels, muffins, rolls, wraps, crackers, cereals, and most other shelf foods, you are eating dead foods. White flour, or most anything white, has been stripped of its bran and germ (which removes the iron, fiber, nutrients, and B-Vitamins), and gives food a longer shelf life. Eating refined foods has gotten us into this mess of chronic disease that permeates our culture. It contributes to insulin resistance, obesity, diabetes, cancer, high blood pressure, and so many other diet related diseases. It's important to pay attention to what you're buying and make sure that you look for "whole grains" in the ingredient list (and no added sugar). "Whole grains" are cereal grains that contain the bran, the germ, and the endosperm of the grain. Most of the nutrients are in the germ and bran. It

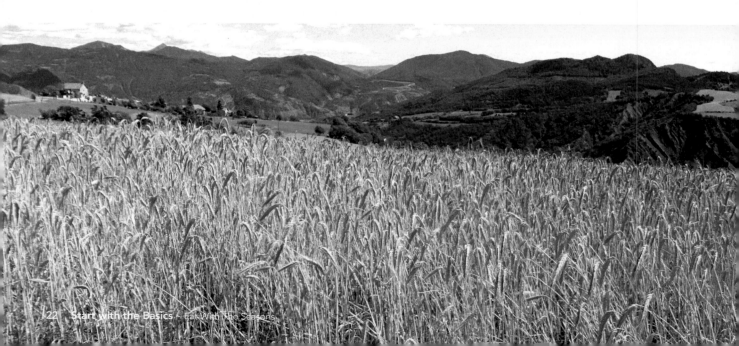

must say "whole wheat" or "whole oat" in the ingredients to actually be a whole grain product. The products we see in the market now are mostly made from "refined grains" and have posed a big problem in our diet. The refining process removes the bran and the hull from the grain, where most of the nutrients and fiber are contained, and leaves us with an unbalanced food high in carbohydrates and sugars.

Although there are many types of grains out there, the cooking and chewing processes are very important in the digestion process. It's important to experiment to see which grains work best for you and you can do this by cooking one grain dish at a time and seeing how you feel after. Does it make you feel satisfied, or do you find yourself feeling bloated and gassy? Some people find that they cannot tolerate many of the grains only to find that they are **gluten-intolerant**. This means that they cannot eat any grains that have gluten in them, namely; wheat, spelt, rye, barley, kamut, farro, triticale. The grains that don't have gluten in them are rice, gluten-free oats, buckwheat, millet, corn, quinoa, and amaranth.

Although whole grains are very healthy for us, not all people can digest them well. This could be a result of several things; it could be the 1.) preparation, 2.) the chewing/digestion, or 3.) allergy.

1. Preparation
Something called phytic acid is present in the hulls of most grains and causes minerals like calcium, magnesium, iron and zinc, to bind with it and render the nutrients non-absorbable in the intestines. This can cause bloating, gas, and discomfort. There are ways to avoid this; soaking grains in water or yogurt, then rinsing and cooking, cooking grains with seaweed, using sprouted grains or sprouted grain flour for cooking, are some options. Soaking (especially grains containing gluten), allows the enzymes to break down and neutralize the phytic acid and this can be helpful in digestion.

2. Chewing/Digestion
Chewing whole grains is the key to better absorption as the digestive process begins in the mouth with the salivary glands. Chewing initiates the release of digestive enzymes in the mouth which help to break down complex carbohydrates and initiate the breakdown into sugars, making the food more alkaline, and helping to make the proteins and nutrients available for absorption. Chewing signals to the stomach that food is on its way and for the stomach to release the acids which will continue the digestive process. People who chew well usually eat less, absorb better, are more relaxed and thinner. Try chewing every mouthful 25 to 35 times.

3. Allergy
Allergies to grains are widespread and getting stronger, especially to wheat. Gluten is an insoluble protein contained in wheat and wheat varieties like kamut and spelt, and in barley, rye, and triticale. It is the protein that gives the doughy consistency to flours. Because it is a very large molecule (and wheat here in the US has been shown to be 25 percent larger than in the past), it is difficult for the digestive system to break it down. Some people cannot. Gluten intolerance or sensitivity means that a person's immune system is intolerant or sensitive to gluten in the diet and displays inflammatory reactions. (A person with celiac disease cannot

tolerate any gluten or alpha gliadin components of the grain, however those who have a sensitivity may be able to tolerate some forms of sprouted or soaked grains). Celiac is usually due to a genetic defect or acquired defect in the intestinal lining. This can cause small intestinal damage and lead to malabsorption and massive nutrient deficiencies, which in turn can lead to any number of disorders including;

- Constipation
- Fatigue
- Joint pain
- Bone pain

- Diarrhea
- Bloating pain
- Gas
- Nausea without vomiting

- Acid reflux
- Leaky gut syndrome
- Arthritis
- Migraines

More severe conditions for someone with undiagnosed celiac disease can lead to anemia, dementia, chronic fatigue, depression, cramps, behavioral learning problems, poor dental health, additional food intolerances, asthma, eczema, bone disease, skin problems and even infertility to name a few. If you suspect intolerance this is not something to put off investigating. The first step is to give up gluten for a 2-week period and see what happens when you reintroduce. *For more information on this see the Resource Chapter.*

Gluten can be found in the whole grains listed previously, but it is also found in many processed foods like broth, breading mixes, condiments, stuffings, imitation seafoods, gravies, sauces, lunch meats, soy sauce, malts, and even nutritional supplements. It is very important to check the ingredient list if you suspect this intolerance. Learn to stick with a whole foods diet to limit your exposure and eat the following if you choose to eat grains at all: rice, corn, soy, potato, tapioca, beans, sorghum, quinoa, millet, buckwheat, arrowroot, amaranth, teff, nut flours, amaranth, popcorn, cornmeal, millet. Millet is gluten free, high in protein, B-Vitamins, calcium, iron, potassium, magnesium, zinc and high fiber. Millet is also a mild thyroid inhibitor and is not recommended if you have a thyroid disease.

How To Cook Whole Grains

Here is an easy to follow guide for cooking whole grains:

1. Measure the grain and check for bugs or unwanted material and rinse in cold water.

2. At this point, you have the option to soak your grains for 1 to 8 hours, which will soften them and make them more digestible as well as eliminate phytic acid. Drain the grains and discard the soaking water.

3. Add grains to recommended amount of water and bring to a boil.

4. A pinch of sea salt, or a piece of seaweed like kombu, may be added to grains to help the cooking process, with the exception of kamut, amaranth and spelt (it interferes with cooking time).

5. Reduce heat, cover and simmer for the recommended time.

COMMON GRAINS:

1 CUP GRAINS	WATER	COOKING TIME (APPROX.)
brown rice	2 cups	60 minutes
buckwheat (kasha)**	2 cups	20 minutes
millet	2 cups	30 minutes
oatmeal (rolled oats)	3 cups	20 minutes
quinoa	2 cups	20 minutes

OTHER GRAINS:

amaranth	2 cups	20 minutes
barley (pearled)	2- to 3 cups	60 minutes
barley (hulled)	2- to 3 cups	90 minutes
bulgur*	2 cups	20 minutes
cornmeal (polenta)	3 cups	30 minutes
couscous	1 cup	5 minutes
kamut	3 cups	90 minutes
oats (whole groats)	3 cups	90 minutes
rye berries	3 cups	2 hours
spelt	3 cups	2 hours
wheat berries	3 cups	60 minutes
wild rice	2 cups	60 minutes

> All liquid measures and times are approximate. It depends a lot on how strong the heat is. It's a good idea, especially for beginners, to lift the lid and check the water level halfway through cooking and towards the end, and also to taste the grains to see if they are fully cooked or starting to burn.

*Bulgur Wheat is made from whole grain red or white wheat that has been parboiled, dried, and ground. It cooks more quickly, is low in fat, and high in fiber and protein.

**You can change the texture of grains by boiling the water before you add the grains. This will keep the grains more separate and less mushy. This is the only way to cook kasha. Do not add kasha to cold water, it will not cook properly. For a softer, more porridge-like consistency, boil grain and liquid together.

FATS IN A NUTSHELL

In my journey to health I have learned so much about fat. I knew that I loved olive oil and good butter but never realized the effects on the body. I also knew that I did not like margarine or anything like it. One of my favorite books is *Fats That Heal Fats That Kill* by Udo Erasmus. This was my bible for learning all the ins and outs and I still don't know everything. Although he can get very technical, he manages to make it very interesting.

So, in a nutshell, how do good fats help us stay healthy? They;

- are necessary for cell growth and division
- regulate vital cell activity
- direct nutrients to the nervous system
- improve concentration
- carry flavor and make food taste good to help the body feel satisfied
- are a carrier for fat soluble vitamins
- A, D, E, & K are metabolized in the body to create body heat, are a source of energy
- free up protein for tissue repair, enhance skin tone, support the immune system
- boost the body's fat-burning ability and improve joint function. Fat is just as important to our survival as proteins, vitamins, minerals and carbohydrates.

Good fats contain Omega 3 and Omega 6 which are Essential Fatty Acids needed by every living cell in the body. Your body cannot make them on its own. You must eat foods that contain these EFAs, and the key is to find the right foods that provide good fats in an optimum ratio for the body. If you are deficient in your EFA's you may experience some of the following symptoms; dry, scaly skin, dry and falling out hair, infertility, gallstones, liver problems, varicose veins, infections, retarded growth, irritability, flightiness and irritability. Check your daily plate and make sure that you are getting a ratio of 40:40:20 (proteins:complex carbohydrates:fats) on a regular basis for optimum health. Be conscious of the type of fats you're eating. Make sure they are not hydrogenated fats or that you have too many saturated fats.

What are hydrogenated fats?
- Highly processed vegetable fats like margarine and shortening
- They are produced with high temperatures
- They are converted to saturated fat by adding hydrogen to the molecules. This changes the configuration of the molecule to a trans fat, which has a drastic effect on its function and properties; it makes the molecules more permeable to carcinogenic substances. It gives the fat a different melting point, chemical activity and enzyme fit, which can impair the natural flow of energy from molecule to molecule within the body. It can worsen the EFA deficiency by interfering with the enzyme systems that transform fatty acids to work in our brain, sense organs, adrenals, and testes. It can interfere with production of prostaglandins, which also interferes with whole body health because the body works to break them down as quickly as it can.

The body metabolizes trans-EFA's for energy, and conserves natural EFA's for more important functions, but the body's break down capacity is limited. If there are too many trans-EFA's and our intake exceeds our limit, disease will manifest. The following are some diseases that have been shown to result from too many Trans-Fatty Acids in the body;

1. Atherosclerosis – which has been shown to increase blood cholesterol up to 15 percent, and increase blood fat levels up to 47 percent. It can increase the size of plaque and the total cholesterol and LDL levels.

2. Cancer – deaths from cancer were 1 in 30 in 1900, and increased to 1 in 4 in 1990. This parallels the increase in our consumption of fats of vegetable origin. There is a close correlation between cancer and increased consumption of hydrogenated and trans-fatty acids.

The other key to healthy fat intake is to keep it fresh. Exposure to heat breaks down the fat and makes it rancid, which is also a source of trans fats. Most fats will break down if exposed to high cooking temperatures (above their smoking temperatures). The key is to know which fats to use when. (Erasmus, Udo)

So what do we eat?

HERE ARE SOME GOOD FAT CHOICES:

- **EXTRA VIRGIN OLIVE OIL:** first cold pressed (expeller pressed), unrefined is best. Good for sautés, cooking at low temperatures (below 132°F), salads, dipping, baking

- **HIGH OLEIC SUNFLOWER OIL & SAFFLOWER OIL:** unrefined, are quite stable for high heat cooking

- **ORGANIC COCONUT OIL:** Good for cooking at all temperatures (has high smoke point), is a very stable fat, good for baking, nice mild flavor, has been shown to be anti-microbial (see Resources, page 248)

- **ORGANIC BUTTER:** Good for cooking and baking

- **GHEE (CLARIFIED BUTTER):** Use as you would butter (can make yourself and store).

- **FRESH NUT AND SEED OILS (AND FLOURS):** Good for eating but not for cooking. Know your source and be sure they are fresh. They turn rancid very quickly if exposed to heat and have a short shelf life. It's best to store in the refrigerator.

- **UNREFINED SESAME OIL:** Use as you would olive oil.

- **GRAPE SEED OIL:** Expeller pressed, good for high heat cooking.

- **PEANUT OIL:** Good for high heat cooking and frying because it has a high smoke point. Another way to use EFA-containing oils in high heat cooking would be to add the vegetables to the pan before putting the oil in. Be sure to keep a watch on the pan.

Many other oils are used as health supplements such as flax seed oil, chia seeds, hemp seeds, evening primrose oil, borage oil, black currant, and fish oils. These are not meant to cook with but as a supplement to the diet.

Easy Solutions & Suggestions

PLANNING IS KEY TO SUCCESS

1. Meal plan for 1 or 2 weeks ahead…keep it simple. Just write down the main meals for 5 out of 7 days in the week.
   a. Make your food list and go shopping
   b. Set aside 1 hour or so per week to prep some of the food so that it's ready when you need it; make a grain, cut up veggies, roast a protein, make beans or legumes

2. Have healthy choices in the house so that you can make and take (see the list of healthy snacks).

3. Think ahead — What is your week going to be like? What do you need to get ready?
   Where are your stress times this week?

4. Drink lots of water and stay hydrated.

5. Make good choices no matter where you are:
   - Convenience stores: Try things like; fruit first, fresh veggies, salads with lean protein like chicken or tuna, yogurt, cottage cheese, seeds and nuts, dried fruit, trail mix free of candy, hard boiled eggs, unsweetened applesauce.

   - The office: This is probably one of the most difficult places for many people. Learn to say no to anything that is not a whole food. Make up your reason and stick to it!!!! So sorry….(sick, disease, allergic, diet, later, whatever!) Then be sure to bring your own. Everyone will love it and you'll start a trend.

   - Restaurant: Start by asking your body what it wants to eat today. Go through the menu and mix and match. It's an art form. Enjoy it! Pick from fresh veggies, whole grains and lean proteins. You choose the restaurant whenever possible. Have a snack before you go, stick to your portions.

   - In the car: Prepare a smoothie to take with you. Leave a supply of your favorites in the car for emergencies. Take along quick to prepare foods from your list.

EASY ON-THE-GO SNACKS

CRUNCH
- apples
- frozen grapes
- rice cakes
- light popcorn or plain popcorn: use coconut oil to pop in a covered pan
- 1 to 2 hard pretzels: the large Bavarian variety
- carrots: particularly the super sweet, organic baby carrots
- crunchy crudités of veggies and dip (humus, tabouleh, vinaigrette, favorite dressing)
- celery and peanut butter or almond butter (use non-hydrogenated peanut butter)
- hummus with whole grain toast, baby carrots, rice crackers

SWEET
- wheatgrass, fresh
- whole fruit organic yogurt and ripe fruit and cacao nibs
- apples and almond butter
- sprouted date bread with jam
- frozen yogurt: freeze your own!
- dried fruit mix and dark chocolate chips or carob chips
- use leftover grains to make sweet porridge: drizzle maple syrup and sprinkle cinnamon, add bananas, heat with fruit juice, etc.
- smoothies: mix whatever you have in the kitchen: fruit, ice, yogurt, carob powder, etc. fruit "ice cream": peel a banana, freeze, blend in a food processor with nuts, berries or raisins and serve; can be put through the screen of a juicer for a creamier consistency
- freshly squeezed fruit juices: make your own and try different combos
- sweet vegetables: yams, sweet potatoes, squashes (acorn, butternut, kabocha) cut into chunks; sprinkle with cinnamon and bake

SALTY
- olives
- pickles
- tabouleh
- hummus
- oysters or sardines
- steamed vegetables with tamari/shoyu
- tortilla chips and salsa or guacamole: try whole grain chips and freshly made salsa or guacamole
- sauerkraut: it will also knock your sweet craving right out!
- fresh lime/lemon juice as seasonings or in beverage
- roasted peanuts or other nuts (make your own trail mix)
- toasted Pumpkin Seeds with herbs and spices

CONDIMENT LIST

Adding condiments to your meals is an exploration in pairings. They add versatility for everyone at the table and can make ordinary recipes come alive. I used to make mixed greens one way and let each person choose which condiments they would like to add to their own plate. Put your condiments on a tray and let family members personalize every meal. Here are some condiments that I can recommend but try adding your personal favorites to the list.

THE BASICS
Garlic powder, ginger, sea salt, gomasio (sesame seeds with sea salt), sea vegetable blends (see Resource page 248 for ordering), ketchup/mustard, sprouts

PEPPERS
Cayenne, chili powder, fresh ground pepper, chili flakes, red pepper flakes, curry powder

OILS, VINEGARS, SAUCES
Extra virgin olive oil, toasted sesame oil, coconut oil, umeboshi paste, umeboshi vinegar (good on grains and beans), balsamic vinegar, apple cider vinegar, tamari soy sauce (gluten-free), shoyu soy sauce, hot sauces, Bragg's amino acids

NUTS & SEEDS
Tahini and other nut butters, nuts like pine, almonds, walnuts, pistachios, raw or toasted pumpkin seeds (see recipe page 43), sunflower or sesame seeds

SWEETENERS
Honey, maple syrup, rice syrup, barley malt, stevia

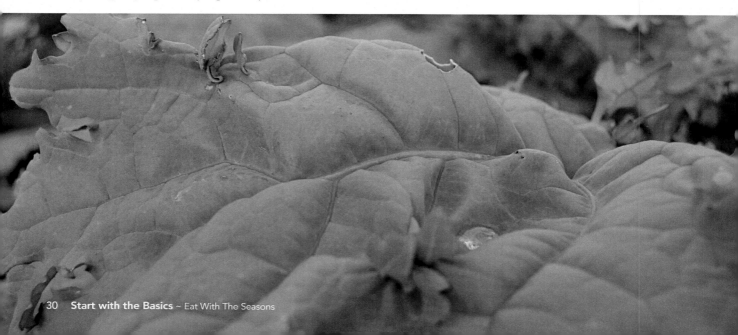

PESTICIDES & YOUR HEALTH

Eating organically grown fruits and vegetables needs to be a conscious decision. The cost to produce this type of food is higher and we have to understand that it will cost us more to purchase at the grocery store. The argument for this choice is a strong one. When we choose organic, we are choosing to have our food free of chemical pesticides, herbicides, antibiotics, hormones, human sewage sludge, and fertilizers that are used on crops to help farmers keep their cost down by not hiring people to weed, harvest and farm. Although there have not been enough studies funded to prove that eating organic is better for your health, there have been many studies linking the chemicals used on our foods (including carcinogens, hormone disrupters, and neurotoxins) to health problems and disease (see Rodale Institute). Even the President's Cancer Panel is recommending that we start to eat food grown without these chemicals and that "the U.S. Government has grossly underestimated the number of cancers caused by environmental toxins", of which these are. In my opinion, we can't afford not to eat organic. This is a subject that needs to be understood because it affects the choices we make every time we eat. Do your own investigating and find out for yourself.

Easy ways to eat organic:

1. Eat seasonal fruits and vegetables from organic producing vendors at the farmer's market. Join an organic fruit CSA (Community Supported Agriculture). Fruit is less expensive when it's in season and comes from a local source. They don't have to pay to ship and they don't waste all the fuel to get it to us.

2. Buy in bulk when it's in season and freeze it. Berries freeze very well. Make applesauce in the fall to eat all winter long.

3. If you shop at the grocery store then choose to buy organically grown fruits and vegetables that are marked USDA Certified Organic. (the PLU code will begin with #9 followed by 4 more numbers)

4. At the very least, focus on foods you eat often and be sure these are organic.

5. Listed below are the 12 most highly sprayed fruits and vegetables and be sure to buy these organically; Peaches, apples, bell peppers, celery, nectarines, strawberries, cherries, kale/collards/spinach and lettuce, grapes, blueberries, potatoes, pears (to see more go to www. foodnews.org)

6. The least sprayed are; onions, avocado, pineapple, mango, asparagus, sweet peas, sweet corn (non-GMO), cabbage, eggplant, cantaloupe, sweet potatoes, grapefruit, mushrooms, kiwi, watermelon.

7. Notice PLU codes as follows;
   - Codes beginning with #3 and #4 are conventionally grown
   - GMO (genetically modified) fruits and veggies have a 5 digit PLU code and begin with #8, ie)-conventional bananas PLU code- 4011
     - organic bananas PLU code- 94011
     - GMO bananas - 84011

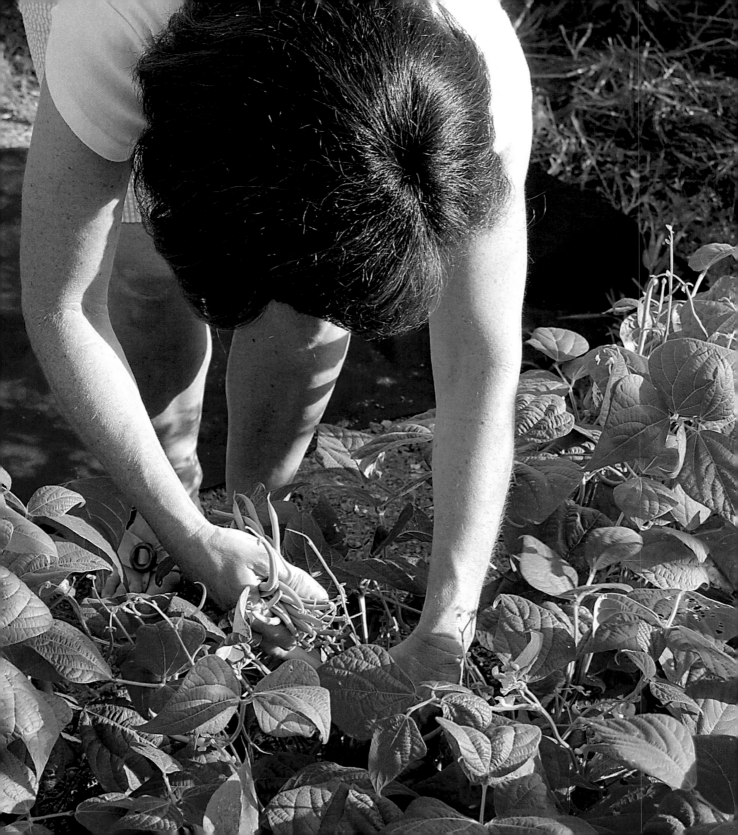

BASIC
RECIPES

3-Grain Pilaf

I learned this great recipe from the Master Chef class I took with Chef Peter Berley. What a great recipe to make at the beginning of the week and use for sides, salads and even in a soup.

- 2 tablespoons olive oil
- ½ cup Scallions or Green Onions, minced (white and tender parts only)
- 1 cup brown basmati rice
- ½ cup millet, soaked and rinsed
- ½ cup quinoa, rinsed
- 3 cups vegetable broth, chicken stock or water
- ¾ teaspoon sea salt
- ¼ cup fresh parsley, chopped, for garnish

▶ Preheat the oven to 350°F.

▶ In a 2- to 3-quart saucepan over medium heat, warm the oil. Add the scallions (and any other vegetables) and sauté for 2 to 3 minutes. Add the rice, millet, quinoa and continue to sauté for 3 minutes more, or until the grains are fragrant.

▶ Add the stock or water and salt. Raise the heat and bring to a boil. Cover the pan and bake in the oven for 30 minutes. (Can also be simmered on stovetop until liquid is absorbed.)

▶ Remove the pilaf from the oven and allow it to rest for 5 minutes. Fluff with a fork, garnish with chopped herbs and serve.

Servings: 6

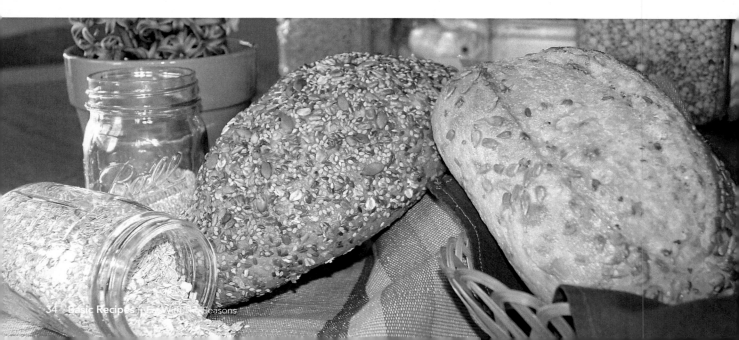

Basic Quinoa With Bay Leaf Infusion

Quinoa is relatively new in our diet in the U.S. but it's been around in South America for ages. It is so easy to make, has a light nutty flavor, and is very high in protein which is a complete protein including all 9 essential amino acids (great for vegetarians and vegans). Quinoa is high in fiber and iron, and a good source of manganese and copper helping to protect the body from free radicals. It makes a great meal with vegetables and beans or add to soups and stews.

- 1 cup quinoa
- 2 bay leaves
- 2 cups water

▶ Rinse quinoa in strainer.

▶ Place in medium saucepan and toast on low flame.

▶ Stir frequently until dry with a nutty aroma.

▶ Add water and bay leaves.

▶ Bring to a boil on high heat.

▶ Reduce heat, cover and simmer on low heat for 15 minutes, set timer. (All liquid will be absorbed.)

▶ Remove bay leaves and serve.

Servings: 6

BASIC VEGETABLE STOCK

This is a recipe for building a stock that can be used for anything. When it calls for water in a recipe you can substitute this and it will give a more complex flavor and add depth to your soups and stews. It can be added to rice to add flavor and you can steam vegetables in it. The best part is that it will also add nutrients to your recipe. I love to make this in quantity and freeze in smaller containers for later use. You can adapt to the seasons by adding the vegetables that are fresh and in season. Kombu can also be added for additional nutrients.

Vegetables to use (preferably organic when possible):
- Onions, garlic,
- Carrots, leek trimmings,
- Celery, potato,
- Chard stems, fresh mushrooms (or broth from dried),
- Scallions, escarole,
- Sea salt, thyme, parsley, bay leaf

For summer stocks add:
- Zucchini and other squash, bell peppers
- Tomatoes, green beans
- Corn cobs, eggplant
- Marjoram, and basil

For winter stocks:
- Celery root, caramelized onions
- Squash and pumpkin seeds
- Roasted garlic and other vegetables
- Dried sage, rosemary

▶ Wash vegetables and coarsely chop. The more vegetables you use, the richer the broth. Heat the olive oil in the pot over medium heat, add the vegetables (except kombu) and cook over high heat for a few minutes, stirring frequently. Add 2 teaspoons sea salt and 2 quarts of water and herbs and bring to a boil. Lower the heat and simmer, uncovered, for 45 minutes or so. Strain.

Yield: 2 quarts

GREENS SAUTÉED IN OLIVE OIL

Green leafy vegetables are the food that is most lacking in the standard American diet. They are so delicious and so easy to make that I just don't understand why this is. I hope this recipe will help to change that for you. Leafy greens, kale in particular, are very high in phytonutrients like Vitamins A, C, E, K, magnesium, potassium, zinc, and easily absorbable calcium. They're high in fiber, they benefit the liver and its cleansing action, contain chlorophyll which helps inhibit viruses and lift mucus. They're energizing and high in antioxidants. The more greens you eat, the less likely you are to eat all the junk food. So jump in!

- 1 bunch kale, rinsed, stems removed and chopped
- ½ bunch Swiss chard (or spinach), or, any combination of your favorite greens like collards, beet greens, spinach
- 2 tablespoons extra virgin olive oil
- 1 medium onion chopped
- 2 cloves garlic, minced
- Fresh lemon juice or umeboshi vinegar, or tamari

▶ Wash, remove stems and chop greens.

▶ Heat olive oil in pan over medium heat, add onion and sauté for about 4 minutes. Add the kale (and collards if using) and stir until they turn bright green. Add about ¼ cup water, cover and steam greens for about 8 minutes. If using, add in the lighter greens like Swiss chard and spinach and cook another 3 minutes.

▶ When greens are cooked, remove cover. Add garlic and sauté for a few more minutes. Sprinkle with lemon juice, umeboshi vinegar or tamari if desired. You could also sprinkle with red pepper flakes and sesame seeds and sea salt if desired. Serve warm.

Servings: 4

MIGHTY MISO SOUP

Another essential staple, this has been known to cure people from whatever ails them. The healing properties of miso are endless. Miso is made from a combination of fermented soybeans and a grain and forms a paste that is high in protein, and loaded with nutrients that support the immune system and the digestive system.

- 1- to 2-inch strip wakame rinsed and soaked 5 minutes in 1 cup of water, until softened
- 1 to 2 cups thinly sliced vegetables of your choice (Daikon, kale, mushrooms)
- 4 to 5 teaspoon barley miso (or other miso if preferable)
- 2 scallions, finely chopped
- 4 to 5 cups spring water

▶ Chop soaked wakame.

▶ Discard soaking water or use on houseplants for a boost of minerals.

▶ Place water and wakame in a soup pot and bring to a boil.

▶ Add root vegetables first and simmer gently for 5 minutes or until tender.

▶ Add leafy vegetables and simmer for 2 to 3 minutes.

▶ Remove about ½ cup of liquid from pot and dissolve miso in the liquid using a whisk. Return it to the pot.

▶ Reduce heat to very low, do not boil or simmer miso broth.

▶ Allow this to cook 2 to 3 minutes.

▶ Garnish with scallions and serve.

Servings: 4

MIXED GREENS PIZZA

This is a great little healthy pizza that can be made very quickly if you substitute a good whole grain pre-made crust, a jar of pesto or tapenade and frozen greens. I love to eat this with olives, goat cheese and anchovies but any toppings will work. Personalize it!

Pizza
- 3 cups fresh spinach or chard, well rinsed, stems removed and large leaves cut into 1-inch wide ribbons
- 3 cups fresh kale, rinsed, cored and chopped
- ½ teaspoon sea salt
- Freshly ground pepper, to taste
- 1 tablespoon extra virgin olive oil
- 1 clove Garlic clove, minced
- ½ cup goat cheese, crumbled
- 2 tablespoons pine nuts
- 6 to 8 Kalamata olives

Pistou
- 2 cloves garlic
- 1 bunch basil leaves, firmly packed
- 1 teaspoon sea salt
- 1 tablespoon extra virgin olive oil

Crust
- 1½ cups whole wheat or spelt flour
- 1 cup cheddar cheese, grated, or shredded
- ½ cup cornmeal, be sure to use the small granules
- 1 teaspoon sea salt
- 4 tablespoons butter, cut into pieces
- 3 tablespoons extra virgin olive oil
- 3 tablespoons ice water

▶ Prepare either a 9x13-inch casserole dish or a large pizza pan or quiche dish by spraying the bottom with olive oil.

▶ Set oven to 350ºF. Bake the crust until it is set but not browned, about 15 minutes. Remove crust from the oven and let cool for a few minutes.

TO PREPARE THE GREENS:
▶ In a sauté pan, steam spinach and kale and Swiss chard with about ¼ cup water for about 5 minutes until wilted. Set aside in a colander and remove the water. In the same pan, put about 1 tablespoon olive oil and add minced garlic and sauté for about 10 seconds then add all the greens back in, salt and pepper, and stir.

TO MAKE THE PISTOU:
▶ In a food processor, put the garlic clove, basil and sea salt, and pulse until minced. Add the olive oil so that the mixture is easily spreadable.

TO ASSEMBLE:
▶ Spread the pistou (or the tapenade) over the bottom of the pizza crust. Layer with the mixed greens. Top with the crumbled goat cheese and pine nuts. You can top with olives if desired.

▶ Bake in the oven until the edges are brown, about 20 minutes (or according to pizza crust instructions). Let it cool for about 10 minutes before cutting or removing from the pan.

Servings: 8

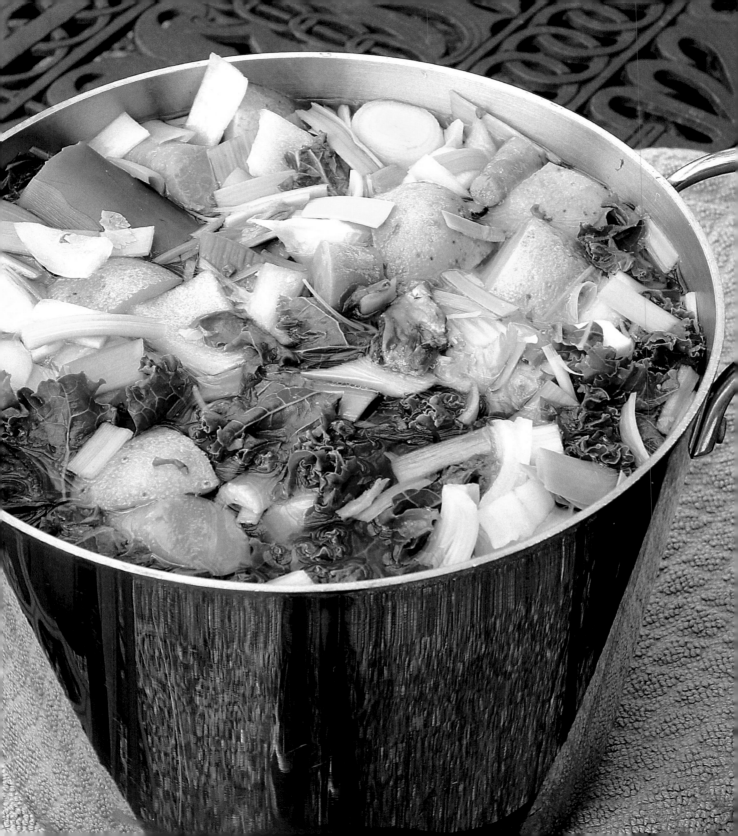

POTASSIUM BROTH

This soup is a staple in our house. I use it as a base for other recipes, but most importantly I use it as a detox and get well broth. When I'm feeling under the weather or need a pick me up, this is what I make. When I've over indulged on vacation (too many lobster rolls), or feel like my diet has been less than normal, this is what I make. When I'm recovering from anything...this is what I love to sip on. It warms my bones and always hits the spot. The addition of the kombu is what does the trick. Try to use organic as much as possible.

- 1 tablespoon olive oil
- 3 to 4 carrots, tops removed, cut up in larger pieces
- 2 potatoes, cleaned and with skin, cut up
- 1 onion, loose paper removed, chopped into quarters
- 3 stalks celery (including leafy part), loosely chopped
- 1 leek, all parts, cleaned and coarsely chopped
- ½ bunch parsley
- 6 garlic cloves, whole
- 1 bunch organic kale, coarsely chopped
- 1 piece kombu or wakame
- ½ head cabbage (optional)
- ½ head broccoli (optional)
- 1 teaspoon miso (optional)
- 2 quarts water

▶ Put olive oil into a Dutch oven and heat to medium. Add the ingredients through leeks and sauté about 3 minutes. Add water and remaining ingredients and bring to a boil. Lower heat to simmer, cover and cook for 45 minutes to 1 hour (or more). Strain and discard solids. Drink the broth warm.

▶ If you are adding miso, be sure to add it after you strain the solids. Do not let the broth come to a boil once the miso is added. Miso has active enzyme properties that make it very good for digestion. These enzymes are destroyed if heated too hot.

▶ Store in the refrigerator, covered, for up to 2 days. Or freeze immediately and use as a stock for soups.

Servings: 16

QUINOA CHOWDER WITH KALE & FETA

Probably one of my most satisfying soups. The added cilantro and feta as toppings make the soup so perfect. This was not even on my radar until I started cooking some of Deborah Madison's recipes from her vegetarian bible book. Although she uses white potatoes and spinach, I love the change I made to sweet potatoes and kale. So satisfying!

- ¾ cup quinoa, rinsed well in a fine sieve
- 2 tablespoons olive oil
- 2 quarts chicken or veggie stock
- 2 garlic cloves, finely chopped
- 1 jalapeño chile, seeded and finely chopped (optional)
- 1 teaspoon ground cumin or to taste
- Sea salt and freshly ground pepper
- ½ pound sweet potatoes, peeled and cut into ¼-inch cubes
- 1 bunch scallions, thinly sliced into rounds
- 3 cups finely sliced kale (or spinach or Swiss chard)
- ¼ pound feta cheese, finely diced
- ⅓ cup chopped cilantro

▶ Put quinoa in a deep sauté pan and toast for several minutes over medium-high heat. Add 2 quarts of chicken or veggie stock and bring to a boil, then lower the heat and simmer for 10 minutes.

▶ While quinoa is cooking, dice the vegetables and crumble the cheese.

▶ Drain quinoa, saving the liquid. Measure the liquid and add water to make 6 cups if needed.

▶ Heat the oil in a soup pot over medium heat. Add the garlic and chile. Cook for about 30 seconds, giving it a quick stir. Add the cumin, 1 teaspoon salt and the potatoes and cook for a few minutes, stirring frequently. Don't let garlic brown.

▶ Add the quinoa water and half the scallions and simmer until the potatoes are tender, about 15 minutes. Add more liquid if necessary to give it a soup consistency.

▶ Add quinoa, kale (or other greens), and remaining scallions and simmer for 3 minutes more. Top with feta and cilantro.

Servings: 6

Roasted Pumpkin Seeds

These are always a hit! Pumpkin seeds are high in zinc, essential fatty acids, and anti-parasitic. They make a great crunchy topping for salads, soups, and sides, and also a great snack to bring along just in case.

- Seeds from 1 large pumpkin or many small, or use 2 cups raw pumpkins seeds or pepitas from the grocery store
- 1 tablespoon olive oil
- 2 teaspoons chili powder
- 2 teaspoons garlic powder
- 1 tablespoon tamari
- 1 tablespoon fresh ground pepper
- 1 tablespoon sea salt

▶ Heat oven to 325°F.

▶ If using fresh seeds from a pumpkin, clean the seeds off and soak them in salted water for about 1 hour. Strain the water when you are ready to bake.

▶ Put seeds into a baggie and add all of the ingredients except salt. Adjust the seasonings according to your liking. Mix all the ingredients together so that they coat the seeds.

▶ Spread seeds onto a cookie sheet and bake for about 30 minutes being careful not to burn. Toss once and bake until lightly browned. Remove and let cool before eating.

Servings: 8

ROASTED ROOT VEGETABLES

One of my favorite comfort food recipes. Because they grow downward and establish a connection with the earth, root vegetables are so grounding and sweet that I find them to be a perfect warming and satisfyingly sweet accompaniment to any dish in the fall and winter. It's such an easy side dish, and a great snack. I like to make lots of extra because the leftover vegetables taste great in soups, omelets, salads, tossed into your favorite grain dish, or just alone. I like to change the herbs or spices according to my cravings or what I am pairing it with. Feel free to change up the vegetables according to your tastes. Use organic whenever possible.

Note: Cut all vegetables same size to allow for even cooking.

- 2 medium organic carrots, scrubbed and julienned into 2-inch pieces
- 2 parsnips, peeled and cut into chunks
- 1 yam or sweet potato, peeled and cut into chunks
- 2 onions, peeled and cut into wedges
- 1 head garlic, pulled apart, keep skins on
- 2 to 3 tablespoons extra-virgin olive oil
- 3 sprigs fresh thyme (or Herbes de Provençe)
- 1 sprig rosemary, leaves chopped
- Freshly ground black pepper and sea salt to taste

▶ Preheat the oven to 350°F.

▶ In a large mixing bowl or a large plastic baggie, place cut up vegetables, olive oil, herbs and pepper and toss well to combine.

▶ Transfer to a shallow baking sheet and bake for 35 to 45 minutes, or until tender. Add sea salt, taste, and adjust the seasonings. Serve warm or at room temperature.

Servings: 8

White Beans a la Provençal

This is a very basic recipe on how to cook dried beans. I love to top the soup with a very flavorful olive oil.

- 1 pound white cannellini or great northern beans, washed and picked over
- 1 tablespoons olive oil
- 1 onion, chopped
- 2 cloves garlic, minced or put through a press
- 5 cups water
- 1 bay leaf
- 6 parsley branches
- Sea salt, to taste
- 1 piece of kombu seaweed
- 1 to 2 cloves garlic, minced
- 1 pound tomatoes peeled and chopped, or, 1 can (28-ounce) diced tomatoes (optional)
- Fresh basil or parsley, to taste, chopped with 1 garlic clove
- Freshly ground black pepper, to taste
- Freshly grated Parmesan cheese
- 1 additional tablespoon olive oil

▶ Soak beans in three times their volume water overnight or for several hours. Drain.

▶ In a large, heavy-bottomed saucepan or casserole heat oil and sauté 1 onion and 2 cloves garlic until onion is tender.

▶ Add beans, bay leaf, parsley, and kombu. Cover with fresh water,

▶ Bring to a slow boil, reduce heat, cover, and simmer 1 hour, or until tender. Be sure to skim off any scum water that rises. When beans are tender and cooked, but not mushy, remove aromatics and kombu. Drain, retaining cooking liquid.

▶ Heat additional olive oil in a wide, heavy-bottomed frying pan or casserole. Add tomatoes (if desired), garlic, salt to taste, and simmer 5 minutes.

▶ Add beans, along with a cup of their cooking liquid, and continue to simmer, covered, 15 minutes. Adjust seasonings. Serve the beans with a little of their broth, in soup bowls with a little extra virgin, unrefined olive oil drizzled over the top, the parsley-garlic mixture and pepper. Grate the cheese over it.

Servings: 8

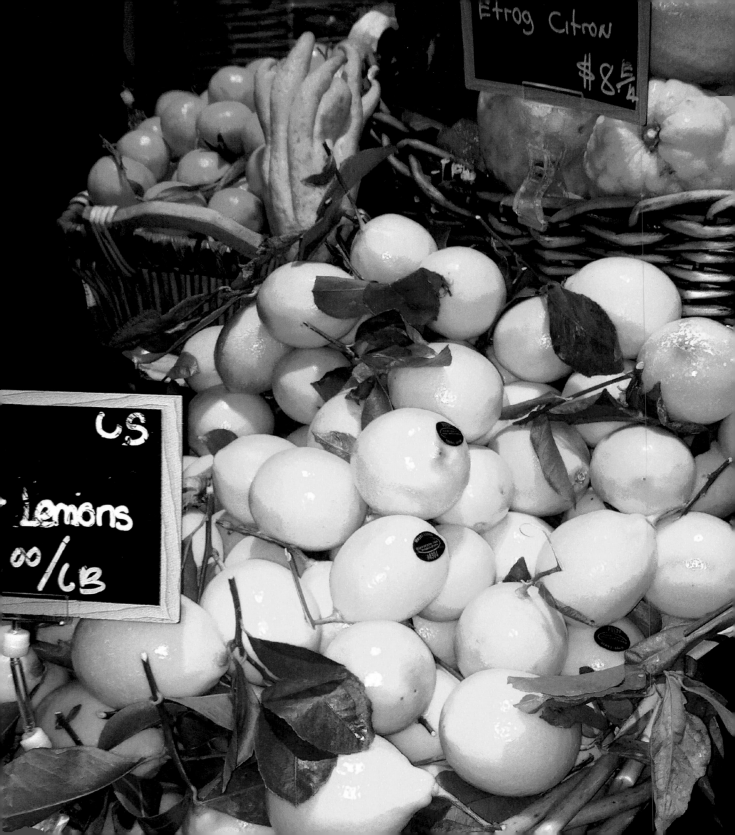

Food & Mood Connection

Primary Causes Of Cravings

The body is truly amazing. The more I learn about our physiology the more awestruck I am at how fine-tuned the body really is. Every little part plays a role in keeping the body balanced and functioning. If left on its own the body will strive to heal itself. We can help our bodies function more smoothly by being aware of the choices we make on a daily basis. Understanding the messages and language of the body is key to identifying the needs, then seeing that they are met. Here are eight primary causes of our cravings.

1. **WATER:** The body doesn't send the message "thirsty" until it's on the verge of dehydration; instead, it often occurs as mild hunger. I find it to be the kind of hunger that I'm not really sure what I want. I look in the refrigerator or pantry and can't really find anything that resolves the craving. So, first thing to do when you get a strange craving is to drink a full glass of water. Wait 5 to 10 minutes and see if you're still hungry.

2. **LACK OF NUTRIENTS:** If the body has inadequate nutrients it will produce odd cravings, for example; inadequate minerals in the diet could produce salt cravings. A generally inadequate nutritional distribution can produce cravings for non-nutritional forms of energy like caffeine, chocolate, sugar. This is where the information on how to deconstruct your cravings comes in handy. If you feel your cravings are due to your diet then source that page and pay attention to what you're eating and how you feel.

3. **SEASONAL:** Often the body craves foods that balance out the elements of the season. For example, often in the spring people crave detoxifying foods like leafy greens or fresh green salads. This can be due to the heavier foods eaten in the winter that the body needs to eliminate to prepare for the warmer season. Light green foods help to energize and cleanse. In the summer people often crave cooling foods like fruit, raw food and ice cream, because of the heat of the weather. It's very interesting how we can trick the body by staying in the AC all summer and the body does not adjust to the heat as well. As fall approaches people tend to crave more grounding foods like squash, root vegetables, and nuts. The weather is getting cooler and soups and stews start to sound so delicious at this time. The cold of winter leaves us craving hot foods and heat producing foods like meat, oil and fat so that we can keep warm through the cold days. As the theme of my book suggests, I am the biggest fan of eating with the seasons so that we help guide the body with our messages of diet.

4. **HORMONAL:** When the body experiences menstruation, pregnancy or menopause its fluctuating testosterone and estrogen levels will often cause strange cravings. How many times do we find women craving chocolate at certain times of the month or during menopausal years. During pregnancy is another time that women crave certain foods. Once again, this is the body speaking its language.

5. **EXTREME FOODS IMBALANCE:** This concept can be very helpful when we are dealing with cravings of the diet. Certain foods have more yin qualities (expanding) while other foods have more yang qualities (contracting). This doesn't necessarily mean that the body expands or contracts, but foods at the opposite poles relieve each other. See the Balancing Chart for a more visual depiction of this concept. The way it

works is, if you are eating foods that are on either extreme, it could cause you to crave the opposite to balance yourself out. For example, if you're eating a diet too rich in sugar (yin), you may find yourself craving meat (yang) or vice versa. If you're eating too many raw foods (yin), like salad and fruit, you may begin to crave extremely cooked (dehydrated) foods like eggs or red meat.

6. **LACK OF NOURISHMENT:** Nourishment comes in many forms, only one of which is food. One of the reasons I include "The Circle of Life" in every chapter is to help you be aware of the other categories that nourish us, and to address these on a regular basis. It's just like your bank account; if you don't keep track and never check the balance you won't know when or where the problems arise. So it is with these other foods that nourish us like, our relationships, our daily work, our exercise routine, or our spiritual life. Are you bored, stressed, or uninspired by your job? Do you lack a spiritual practice that gives you a greater sense of being? Are you in a relationship that is toxic to your soul? You may find yourself experiencing emotional eating or eating for entertainment just to fill the void of the lack of these other nourishing foods in your life. One of the activities you can do to help differentiate between whole foods and other nourishing foods, is to create a list of "Things That Nourish Me". Make a list of 1 to 10 things, other than food, that nourish you in other ways. Sometimes when we think we're hungry it's really just our feelings calling out to us for attention. Feeding these feelings with something other than food can help to end the urge and bring nourishment to the soul. It can be anything from going for a walk or taking a bath, to reading a book or getting a massage. What nourishes you?

7. **COMFORT CRAVINGS:** Sometimes you'll find yourself craving something you've eaten in the past; either foods similar to what your ancestors ate, foods that you ate as a child, or something you recently ate. I once found myself craving Spaghettios ("that neat little treat you can eat with a spoon"), and I couldn't for the life of me figure it out. Then I realized that I used to eat this at a good friend's house when I was young and it always carried such fond memories with it. Needless to say, I decided to try some and it just did not do the trick! A good way to reconstruct these cravings is to first ask yourself what it is you are craving. It could be nostalgia for a time less difficult. Maybe you are overdue with communicating with someone and you need to touch base. Maybe you just want to relive some of the fond memories without eating the food. If the craving comes often and the food is not very healthy, you could either eat a healthier version of your ancestral or childhood foods, or just eat just a small amount of the "real thing".

8. **SABOTAGE AND ADDICTION EATING:** Sometimes when things are going just a little too well, we sometimes feel the need to sabotage ourselves by craving foods that throw us off our track. It gives us an escape from our power and potential. The idea is that if we continue to do well and feel good, it may lead us to new heights and new power that we are not sure we know what to do with. It can be a little unsettling and uncomfortable to move out of our comfort zone so thus we sabotage ourselves by eating foods that throw us into imbalance, creating some chaos thus giving us reason to regress.

WHAT ARE YOU CRAVING & WHY?

What is the quality of your cravings? What do you choose to eat? Are you eating extreme foods? Use this simple chart to help you get on your way to deconstructing your cravings. Your body strives to keep balance every second of the day. When you are craving something it is your body sending you a message. That's how it communicates with you and you need to listen. As you pay attention you will become better at discerning the hidden messages of your cravings. Get used to asking "What does my body want and why?"

- Craving salty foods? Maybe you need minerals like sea salt, vegetables, and leafy greens.

- Craving bitter, like coffee and beer? This could be a sign of stagnancy. Try adding in fresh leafy greens like arugula and watercress. Do a cleanse for your liver.

- Craving pungent like pickles and vinegar? This could mean that you need to spark the digestive tract. Try adding in ginger, scallions, and leeks.

- Craving spicy and hot? Your blood could be thick from dead foods like refined foods, or from a diet of heavy fats and meats, and a slow circulation. This can often occur after the winter season. Try adding spices like cayenne pepper, onions, garlic, and celery.

- Craving things with texture? Maybe you're eating too many refined products like bread, crackers, and flour products. You could be stuck and irritable. Or it could be from eating from the creamy texture of too much ice cream or milk products. Add more olive oil and good fats to the diet.

- Craving moist or liquid? Maybe you're eating too many salty or dry foods, or you could be dehydrated from not enough water or lack of watery foods like fruits and vegetables.

- Craving crispy and dry? With the water craze that's going on maybe you're drinking too much liquid and you need to pay attention. If you're feeling tight, constipated, tense or stressed… take a look at your exercise regime and the extreme foods that are in your diet. Maybe you are eating too much protein or rushing your schedule. Try taking time to do breathing exercises on a daily basis and add in lots of leafy green vegetables.

- On the other hand, if you're feeling drowsy, dizzy, confused, weak, or hungry… consider that you could be hypoglycemic. If this is the case then you must see your doctor right away. Otherwise you may be in a period where you are eating too much sugar, alcohol and refined foods. Time to add in more whole grains and fish/poultry/beans.

BALANCE CHART

The basis for this chart comes from the book by Kristina Turner called *The Self-Healing Cookbook*. I have often sourced this chart to resolve my dietary cravings when they occur. It can be used as a quick fix for something like a headache, or for a broader overview of what might be happening in the diet. The middle of the chart is where 80 percent of your diet (from fruits and nuts to fish/poultry) is best chosen in order to prevent imbalances.

FROM EXTREMELY EXPANSIVE TO BALANCING:

- alcohol and chemicals
- sugar and coffee
- honey and spices
- butter and oil tropical fruits
- potato and tomato

- **local fruit and nuts**
- **tofu, leafy greens, seeds**
- **root vegetables and winter squash**
- **beans and sea vegetables**
- **whole grains**
- **fish**

 80% of your diet

FROM BALANCING TO EXTREMELY CONTRACTIVE:

- poultry
- cheese
- red meat
- miso and tamari
- eggs
- salt

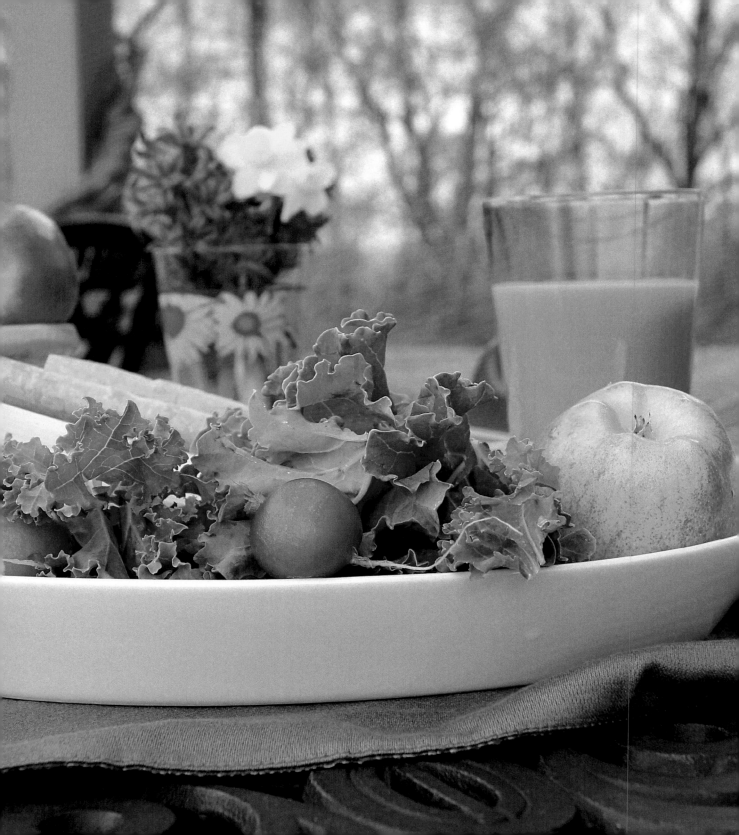

FOOD & MOOD CONNECTION

I have learned that a connection to our food source can have a profound affect on how we think, the decisions we make, and the joy we discover in our lives. What we choose to eat and the mindfulness with which we eat it affects us. When we're eating fast food cheeseburgers with french fries and milkshakes we feel differently and make different choices then when we're eating salads, broccoli and wild caught salmon. I'm including this easy to use chart that was developed by myself and a co-worker for use with our weight management groups. It's a great way to change things up when your mood needs an adjustment.

PROCEDURE:

- **FEELING:** Overwhelmed, afraid, cold, worried, over sensitive, self conscious, **but want to feel** relaxed, content, warm, calm, centered, acceptance.
- **DO THIS:** yoga and meditation, walking, jogging, weight lifting.
- **COOK THIS:** miso soup, cooked sweet potato, cooked greens and brown rice with sesame oil, cooked root vegetables and winter squashes, spices, bananas, oranges, almonds, oats with cinnamon or maple syrup.

- **FEELING:** Impatient, frustrated, tense, dramatic, **but want to feel** patient, decisive, relaxed, playful.
- **DO THIS:** walking, jogging, swimming, yoga and meditation, weight lifting.
- **COOK THIS:** barley, white beans, cooked bitter greens, raw vegetables, sunflower seeds, quinoa, salad and vegetables, apples, pears, pineapple.

- **FEELING:** Stuck, sad, depressed, **but want to feel** energized, content, clear.
- **DO THIS:** movement, walking fast, running, dancing, biking, spinning, weight lifting, power yoga, meditation.
- **COOK THIS:** brown rice, lentils, greens, miso, onion, ginger, sprouts, dried fruit.

THE CIRCLE OF LIFE

The **Circle Of Life** is a tool that I have used frequently for myself, for clients, and other workshop groups. There are many versions but this is the one I learned at The Institute for Integrative Nutrition and I find it to be very useful. It's a tool to help identify where you are at the moment and what areas in your life might need attention now. I like to use it seasonally to help pull my attention and intentions to areas of my life that need it. I have inserted one per season for your use. It's hard to pay attention to every aspect of our lives at all times so we tend to turn them on and off depending on events or transitions taking place in our lives and the stress levels that accompany them. Sometimes we only operate in crisis mode, putting out fire after fire, but never recuperating and rejuvenating afterward. This circle is an attempt to address those areas of importance before they rage into out-of-control fires and cause stress and disease. The purpose is to look at each segment of the circle and draw a dot in each category based on how satisfied you are at this moment with that area of your life. It has nothing to do with comparisons to others and societal measurements; simply with your satisfaction at this moment in time. Once you have placed a dot in each category, with the outer edge being the most satisfied and inner circle the least, you connect the dots to see your current circle of life. Although we usually know where we need to focus our attention, this makes a glaring illustration for us. I then ask people to pick the top three areas, circle them and write them down at the bottom of the page. Ask yourself, what's one thing I can do this season to move me in a more joyful direction for this category. Write it down and get started by meditating on the action each day.

"Attention energizes and intention transforms... The quality of intention on the object of attention orchestrates an infinity of details to bring about the intended outcome." – Deepak Chopra

As you fill out the circle, here are some thoughts to ask yourself...

- **RELATIONSHIPS:** Are they fulfilling? Are they draining you? Do you have open communication? Anything toxic?

- **SOCIAL LIFE:** Do you have a good social circle that meets your needs. Are they fun? Do you have deep connections? Can you trust them? Are you meeting new people? Do you want any of these?

- **JOY:** Most important of all, are you finding this in your daily life? In what areas? What might be draining your power and joy? Why?

- **SPIRITUALITY:** Are you aware of a connection with the universe, higher self, higher power? Do you devote any time to this area? Do you pray or meditate? Are these important to you?

- **CREATIVITY:** Are you expressing yours? In what way? Is it enough? Where can you find this expression if not?

- **FINANCES:** How wealthy are you and how do you feel about this at the moment? Do you have savings/cash flow? Is this area infringing on other areas?

- **CAREER-JOB-WORK:** Is what you do most of the day satisfying to you? How are you performing in this area? Are you fulfilled? Are you energized and passionate? Does it work for you?

- **EDUCATION:** Are you achieving your highest potential for now? Are you growing/learning in ways you enjoy?

- **HOME COOKING:** What percentage are you cooking? Are you eating whole foods? Is your diet in balance? Are you making healthy choices no matter where you eat? Are you addicted to anything?

- **PHYSICAL ACTIVITY:** Do you get enough? Are you energized? Do you exercise regularly and have a plan? Does it make you happy?

- **HEALTH:** In general how is your diet, lifestyle? Do you sleep well and enough? Are you focused? Are you sick?

- **HOME ENVIRONMENT:** Is it relaxing, stress free, satisfying, joyful, and peaceful for you? Are there any aspects that drain your power? Do you rejuvenate here? Do you have personal space? I like to end by having you ask yourself...What have you been putting off? Why? Are you giving back? How?

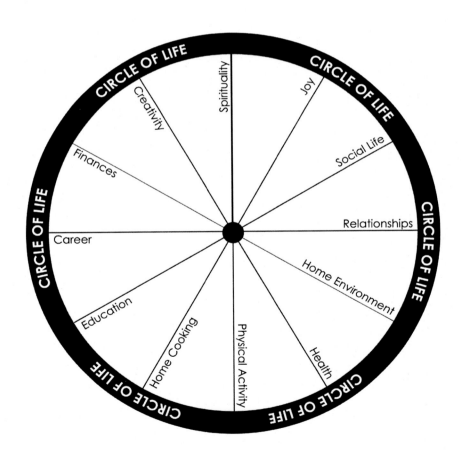

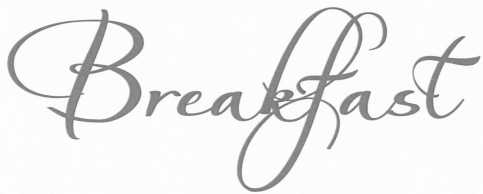

Breakfast

"Eat breakfast like a king, lunch like a prince,
and dinner like a pauper…"
– ADELLE DAVIS

Start Strong – Stay Strong

Although I am not a "big" breakfast eater, I really need to eat my breakfast to get me started on the right foot for the rest of the day. I have done many breakfast experiments trying to decide what works best for me and I realize that everyone is different in their needs. (If you haven't tried doing a breakfast experiment for yourself you might want to consider it because it's quite an eye-opener.) Not only are our bodies different but so are our schedules. If I had to leave the house every morning at 6 a.m., I would no longer want to eat eggs regardless of whether they are good for me or not. It's truly a matter of figuring out what works for you and your schedule. I realize that I have many rituals that I really love. My morning ritual is one of them. It's quite simple, and has changed with the years, but it works for me. I like to be quiet in the morning and I have a process of making coffee, drinking water with lemon, doing my stretches, and some meditations and readings that get me centered for the day. I accomplish this ritual with much mindfulness and joy and I realize that the difference between a ritual and a rut is all in the mindfulness and joy in which it is carried out. The most mundane rituals can be joyful when I pay attention. No doubt, I have many days when I just want to be done with my tasks and my mind is on my "busy" schedule and the list of things to be done. On these days I don't feel the exhilaration and joy of my rituals. What a waste!

On the other end there are the health reasons that make breakfast the most important meal of the day for me. If I fuel myself with a balanced breakfast (and I have many suggestions for that), it gives me long and short term energy, gets my metabolism moving, keeps me satiated until lunch and I get my work done with a satisfied feeling. It tells my body that it is not going to starve today so it does not have to store fat. Studies show that it's best to eat within an hour or so of rising. Reason: at night 80 percent of your glycogen stores (digested carbohydrates) are used up. Even if you work out on an empty stomach you will use up the rest of the 20 percent and tap into your lean muscle mass rather than your fat stores (Jillian Michaels). It's best to have some trail mix and maybe half of an apple before exercising so that you use this energy instead. It's also very important to rehydrate as soon as you rise because the body dehydrates nightly doing all its work. Try to wake up each day to room temperature water with lemon. The lemon is great for activating the digestive system. Skipping breakfast or choosing an "empty" breakfast contributes to: less effective concentration, foggy thinking, low blood sugar causing irritability and lack of energy, poor food choices throughout the day, and over eating at night. In studies it has been shown that women who skip breakfast are 4½ times more likely to become obese. People who never eat breakfast are more likely to develop type 2 diabetes. In a study in Pediatrics (March 2008), they tracked adolescents for five years and found that those who ate more breakfast had a lower BMI and weighed less at the age of 20. If you're not waking up hungry it might be a good idea to look at your dinner habits. If you eat a late dinner or snack before bed, you are not giving your body the proper time it needs to digest, burn fat, and release the growth hormones it needs. A good 9 to 10 hours of "fasting" is ideal according to many experts. Then you'll wake up feeling hungry and ready to "break the fast". A good rule for me is that I don't eat after 9 p.m. — especially carbs (unless of course I'm out at a really good restaurant or celebrating!!).

MY THOUGHTS ON BREAKFAST EATING: Eat something with protein, fat and carbohydrates each morning in a portion size that satisfies without making you feel too full.

THE BREAKFAST EXPERIMENT

This is a great little exercise to figure out what kinds of foods work best for you in the morning. Explore eating a different breakfast every day for one week. Make a note of how you feel right after eating, and again 2 hours later. Try to sit quietly after you eat and note energy levels, moods, and physical symptoms affected during your morning. You may discover that you are unusually sensitive to certain foods (even if they are "good for you" foods). With the prevalence of gluten sensitivity and food allergies so common nowadays, this is a good way to tune in to what your body has to say and take notice.

DAY 1: scrambled eggs (or tofu) with spinach and potatoes.

DAY 2: whole grain toast, coffee/tea or other beverage

DAY 3: oatmeal with milk (rice or almond if preferred), raisins, 3-ounces plain yogurt, beverage

DAY 4: boxed cereal with a milk, beverage

DAY 5: fruit, yogurt, beverage

DAY 6: muffin, beverage

DAY 7: fresh vegetables

Each day for one week, make note of:

- what you eat
- when you eat it
- how you feel right after eating
- how you feel 2 hours later
- when you feel hungry again
- If you find this too difficult to do in one week, try spreading it out over a few weeks time and pick one or two days in the week that you experiment.

Almond Banana Smoothie

This is one of my favorite recipes to turn to when I'm in the mood for ice cream but don't want to eat all the sugar, dairy and fat found in ice cream. I love the crunch of the nibs. It can be a good breakfast choice because it's quite filling. I freeze bananas in pieces to make this a little thicker.

- 1½ cups almond milk, cold
- 1 tablespoon cocoa powder
- 1 tablespoon cacao nibs
- 2 tablespoons agave nectar or maple syrup
- 1 teaspoon healthy oil (flax, pistachio, olive)
- ½ banana or more to taste
- 1 tablespoon almond butter or peanut butter (optional)

▶ Put all ingredients in blender and whip up a healthy and filling milkshake.

Servings: 1

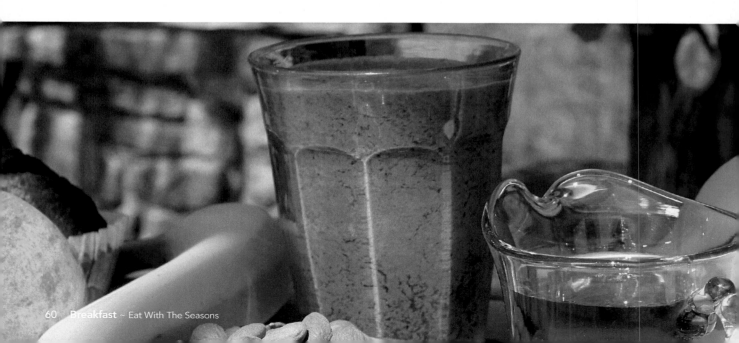

APPLESAUCE BRAN MUFFINS

These are the best muffins for breakfast or snack or even lunch. High in fiber and protein, but moist and tasty. One of these muffins along with my green smoothie is the perfect breakfast for me.

- 1½ cups spelt flour
- 1 cup oat bran
- 2 teaspoons baking powder
- ½ teaspoon baking soda
- 1 teaspoon cinnamon
- 1 teaspoon allspice
- ½ teaspoon nutmeg
- 1 teaspoon sea salt
- 2 tablespoons wheat germ
- 1 egg, beaten
- ½ cup Pure Maple Syrup
- ½ cup dates, pitted and chopped
- 1 tablespoon molasses
- 1 tablespoon olive oil
- 1¼ cups applesauce with no sugar added

▶ Preheat oven to 350°F. Fill muffin tin with the little paper cups.

▶ Mix the flour, bran, baking powder, baking soda, spices, salt, and wheat germ in a large bowl.

▶ Make a well in the center and add the egg, maple syrup, and molasses. Blend well. Gradually stir in the applesauce and mix thoroughly. Fold in the dates.

▶ Fill the muffin mold with about ⅔ cup of batter per muffin. Bake for 25 to 30 minutes, until the tops are light brown.

▶ Store in plastic bags after cooled, or wrap individually and freeze.

Servings: 12

Avocado-Tomato-Cheese Toastie

The first time I ever ate one of these was when I was visiting my daughter in Australia. We went to a simple breakfast place and they had the best little open-faced meals that they called "toasties". We could pick from many toppings that were fresh and healthy. This was one of my favorites. Make up your own with simple foods you love.

- 1 piece sprouted grain bread, toasted
- ½ avocado, peeled and sliced
- ½ tomato, sliced
- 1 tablespoon plain yogurt
- ¼ cup cheese such as feta, goat, Gouda

▶ Toast the bread. Spread the yogurt on top, place the tomatoes then avocados on top. Sprinkle with salt and pepper or condiments of your choice. Top with some cheese and stick under the broiler for about 1 minute and a half. Enjoy!

Serving: 1

Baked Oats Granola

This is a nice make ahead breakfast that you can bring with you on the road for those times when you don't have time to sit and eat breakfast. If you add it to some plain yogurt, and berries, or add almond milk then you have a yummy complete breakfast.

- 6 tablespoons butter
- 4½ cups old-fashioned rolled oats
- 1½ cups shredded coconut
- 1¾ cups sliced almonds (6 ounces)

- 6 tablespoons honey or real maple syrup
- ¾ teaspoon ground cinnamon
- ½ teaspoon salt
- 1 cup raisins

▶ Put butter into 9x13x2-inch baking pan and melt in oven at 350°F, about 5 minutes. Remove from oven and add rolled oats, coconut and almonds. Drizzle with honey and sprinkle with cinnamon and salt.

▶ Return to oven and bake 25 to 30 minutes, stirring frequently, until almonds are toasted and mixture is golden brown. Remove from oven; stir in raisins. Cool completely, stirring once or twice, and store in airtight container.

Servings: 12 / Yield: 2 quarts

BLUEBERRY BUCKWHEAT MUFFINS

I found a version of these muffins in a magazine and proceeded to alter the flours, sweeteners, and oils to load them with more nutrients. Here I use spelt and buckwheat flours. Buckwheat is gluten free and helps to strengthen blood vessels and reduce blood pressure due to "rutin", a bioflavonoid found in this grain. It is high in fiber, as is spelt, and in magnesium. If toasted, buckwheat is known as "kasha". I love to have one of these muffins for breakfast. Blueberries are rich in manganese, a mineral essential to healthy ligaments, and high in antioxidants.

- 1½ cups spelt flour
- ½ cup buckwheat flour
- 2 tablespoons wheat germ
- 2 tablespoons oat bran
- 2 teaspoons baking powder
- ¼ teaspoon baking soda
- ½ teaspoon sea salt
- 2 large eggs
- ¾ cups pure maple syrup
- ¼ cup coconut oil, melted or at room temperature
- 1 cup unsweetened applesauce
- 1½ teaspoon lemon zest
- 1 teaspoon vanilla
- ¾ cup kefir or plain yogurt
- 1½ cups blueberries (frozen or fresh) (if using frozen blueberries, add ¼ cup more spelt flour)
- ⅓ cup sunflower seeds

▶ Preheat oven to 400°F. Grease 12 regular-size muffin tins or line with foil baking cups.

▶ In a medium bowl, whisk the flours, baking powder, baking soda, sea salt, oat bran and wheat germ.

▶ In a large bowl, whisk the eggs, maple syrup, and oil until well blended and slightly frothy. Whisk in the applesauce, lemon zest, and vanilla. With the whisk, stir in about half the flour mixture, then half the kefir (yogurt). Repeat with the remaining flour and kefir, stirring until well incorporated. Gently fold in the blueberries.

▶ Divide the batter among the muffin cups, filling them to the top. Tap the pan on the counter to remove any air bubbles. Sprinkle each muffin with about ½ teaspoon of sunflower seeds. Bake for about 20 to 30 minutes, until a toothpick inserted in center comes out clean.

▶ Let muffins cool on a rack for 15 minutes. They taste best warm. To store, cool completely and store in an airtight container at room temperature, or wrap individually and freeze for up to 3 months.

Servings: 12 / Yield: 12

BUCKWHEAT PUMPKIN SPICE MUFFINS

These muffins are moist and spicy and gluten-free. I like them for breakfast but they also make a great snack.

- 2 eggs
- ¾ cup cooked pumpkin, mashed (or canned)
- 2 tablespoons coconut oil
- ⅔ cup applesauce
- 3 tablespoons maple syrup
- 1 tablespoon molasses
- 1 cup buckwheat flour
- ¼ cup soy flour
- 1 tablespoon baking powder

- ¼ teaspoon sea salt
- 1 teaspoon baking soda
- 2 teaspoons cinnamon
- 1 teaspoon ginger
- ½ teaspoon ground cloves
- ½ teaspoon nutmeg
- ½ cup raisins
- 1¼ cups chocolate chips – good quality, dark (optional)

▶ Grease 12 regular size muffin cups or line with foil baking cups.

▶ In a mixing bowl or food processor, blend together the eggs, pumpkin, oil, applesauce, maple syrup, and molasses.

▶ In another bowl, mix together the flours, baking powder, baking soda, salt, spices and raisins. Add dry mixture to wet ingredients and blend. Stir in chocolate chips.

▶ Bake for 15 to 20 minutes or until knife inserted comes out clean.

Servings: 12 / Yield: 14

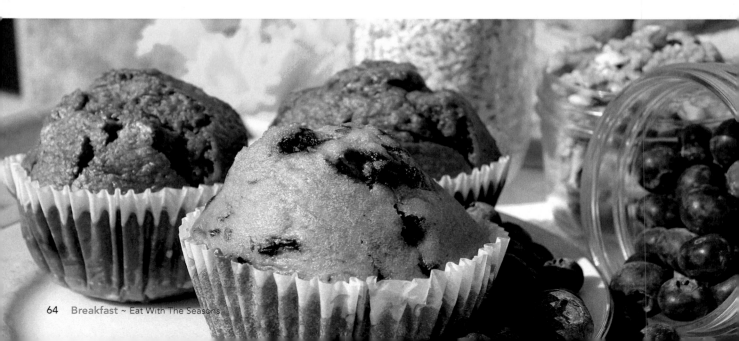

CROCKPOT BREAKFAST

Although whole grains take much longer to cook than the refined quick type, they are well worth the trouble it takes. Whole grains contain all the fiber, minerals, fats, and proteins needed to fuel the body for a good start to the day. This recipe helps make things easier by cooking everything in the crockpot so it's all ready to eat in the morning. Add some cinnamon to make the whole house smell delicious when you come into the kitchen.

- ½ cup short grain brown rice
- ½ cup millet
- ½ cup steel cut oats
- 8 cups water
- ½ cup (or more) dates, raisins and other dried fruit, pitted and chopped
- 1 teaspoon vanilla
- 1 teaspoon lemon juice

▶ Prepare the night before.

▶ Thoroughly wash all the grains and drain.

▶ Add all ingredients into crockpot and stir to mix.

▶ Cook on low all night.

▶ In the morning, stir and serve with almond milk, cinnamon and maple syrup.

Servings: 6

Slow Cooker Steel Cut Oats

I like to store the extra in individual serving sizes to pull out for breakfast each morning.

- 1 cup steel cut oats
- 4 cups water (or use ½ water, ½ almond milk)
- Cinnamon, to taste
- Raisins, bananas, strawberries, etc, to taste

▶ Combine oats and water (and almond milk if you are using), in a slow cooker. Add cinnamon, if desired. Cook for 7 to 8 hours on low setting.

▶ Wake up in the morning, add your other things to your oatmeal and enjoy. Refrigerate any leftovers.
    Servings: 4

Steel Cut Oats with Cinnamon, Raisins & Maple Syrup

On those chilly winter days I love the taste of these hearty steel cut oats with the cinnamon and the sweet flavor of real maple syrup. Whole grains are perfect for providing balanced energy all morning long because the body absorbs them slowly. They also contain fiber and B Vitamins and help to ward off hunger and cravings. It works for me!

- 1 cup steel cut oats, rinsed well and soaked overnight if desired (for speedier cooking)
- 3 cups water
- Pinch sea salt
- 1 teaspoon cinnamon
- ⅓ cup raisins
- 4 tablespoons real maple syrup, or more to taste
- 1 tablespoon milk, like almond, rice, goat or even yogurt

▶ Bring the water and salt to a boil over medium heat. Slowly add the rinsed oats to the water and stir. Let cook for about 10 to 15 minutes being sure that all the water is absorbed and adding more water if it evaporates too quickly. The longer you cook it the easier it will be to digest.

▶ Remove from the stove and add cinnamon, raisins and maple syrup. Serve the portion that you will eat that day, adding some rice or almond milk if desired.

▶ Take the leftover oats and add some rice milk to make it somewhat more liquid. Store this in the refrigerator until tomorrow when all you will have to do is heat it up.

    Servings: 4 / Yield: 2 cups

Spelt-Sunflower Pancakes

These are the only pancakes I have found made from whole grains that actually taste good. I love the rich flavor of the spelt flour and bran.

Dry Mix — can be made ahead
- 4 cups spelt flour
- ½ cup sunflower seeds
- 1 tablespoon oat bran
- 1 tablespoon wheat germ
- 4 teaspoons baking powder
- 2 teaspoons baking soda
- 2 teaspoons sea salt
- 1 teaspoon ground cinnamon

To make Pancake Batter mix together;
- 2 large eggs
- 1¼ cups buttermilk, plus more if needed
- 2 tablespoons olive oil or coconut oil
- 1 teaspoon real maple syrup

▶ To make dry mix; combine all ingredients in a large bowl. Set aside 1½ cups and divide remainder and store in resealable plastic bags for later use.

▶ To make pancakes; beat eggs in large bowl. Whisk in buttermilk, syrup and oil. Add Dry Mix and stir to combine. Do not over-mix. Add more buttermilk if batter is too thick.

▶ Heat griddle or skillet over medium heat. Coat lightly with oil. Pour on ¼ cup batter and cook.

Servings: 12

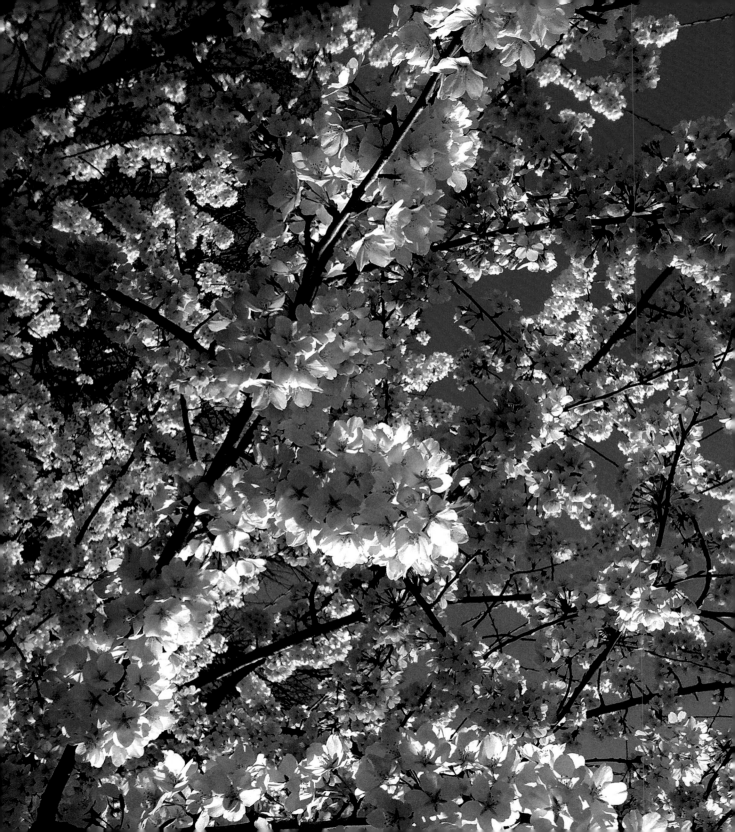

Spring

"Eat food. Not too much. Mostly plants."
– Michael Pollan

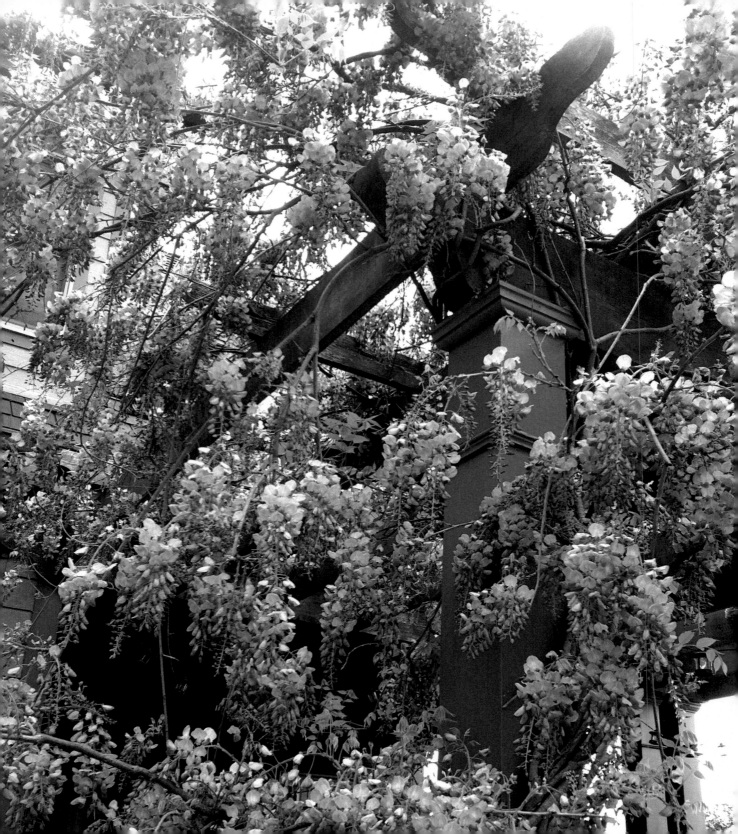

SHIFTING INTO SPRING

At long last SPRING!!! My season of inspiration and renewal. After the calm and quiet of winter we now flow into a burst of life. I always know that spring is here when I hear the first sound of the spring peepers coming from the ponds and woods nearby. It's music to my ears and brings a smile to my face. The earth is born again with new life and activity; green shoots appear from the earth again, the grass turns a rich green, the soil has that earthy, damp smell, the redbud sends out its pink flower to add a splash of pink to the grey woods, and crocuses appear on sunny walkways, fruit trees begin their glorious show of colorful succession; from pear to cherry to plum to apple, like a parade of color. The weather teases us with warm days then lapses into windy, cold again. I love to find time to sit on the sunny side of my house, where the wind is blocked, and get as much sunshine as possible. It always feels so good...like my body is craving the Vitamin D and pulls in every ray of sunshine it can.

My thoughts on shifting… THINK GREEN, DETOX

The spring equinox occurs on March 21 and this is when there is equal amounts of day and night. This is the time to start easing into green foods that are bitter and cleansing. Add fresh sprouts to your green salads along with chives, green onions, watercress, and parsley. Raw foods can have a cooling effect on the body and help us to feel lighter. This could be a good time to try some of the sea vegetables, cereal grasses like wheatgrass, or micro-algae like spirulina. These have all been shown useful for liver and blood health. I love to take time for a gentle detox each spring to rid my body of the heavy foods of winter. It helps energize my body and give me more vitality. Although there are many levels of detoxing, I stick to a few days of drinking juices and broths made from fresh fruits and vegetables. I add in fresh raw salads and cooked grains and legumes after a couple of days. I try to schedule this for a few days when I can take time to walk outside, and carve out some quiet time to reflect and rest. It's a wonderful rejuvenation for spring that helps re-set my metabolism for the warmer weather to come. A spring detox is a great time to air out negative thoughts and emotions, spring clean our living space and make room for fresh air. Spring is the time for a new plan, a fresh start, and a season to let your dreams blossom.

Spring Seasonal Plan

BREAKFAST OPTIONS: What spring options would you like to add to your breakfast routine? This is a good time to begin lightening things up. Plain yogurt with berries and nibs, smoothies, sprouted grain toast, homemade muffins, could be some good choices. Write down your spring breakfast choices here:

_____

SNACK OPTIONS: Add in lots of fresh berries, fresh spring greens with seeds, crunchy radishes, snap peas, and broccoli. What are your spring snack choices? Write them here:

_____

LUNCH: What are your all time favorites? Now add in some choices that are seasonal. As the days get warmer it's time to lighten up the diet with more green salads, lots of fresh vegetables and berries, lighter, broth type soups. Write your lunchtime choices here:

_____

MENTAL RECIPE FILE: Go through your mental recipe file and think back to meals you like to make in the spring. Which old stand by's would you like to keep that are still working for you? Write those here;

_____

NEW SPRING OPTIONS: Now take a look at the menus in this chapter. Which recipes sound good enough that you would like to try adding to your mental recipe file? Choose 3 to 5 and these are the recipes that you will be working with this spring. Make them your own by working with the ingredients to create a meal that is satisfying to your needs. Write the recipe names here:

_____

_____

SPRING EXERCISE: What changes are you going to make to your SPRING routine to help you flow with the season? Have you been intending to try a new class, sport, game? Why not put it in your schedule and try it out? If you have been exercising inside all winter, this is a nice time to move outside and enjoy the warming sunshine and refill your Vitamin D tank. Write your exercise commitments here:

_____

_____

_____

YOUR SPRING CIRCLE OF LIFE

Your life at this moment is a direct result of your actions over the last months and years.

This exercise will help you to discover which nourishment you are missing most. The Circle of Life has ten sections. Look at each section of the circle and place a dot on the line to designate how satisfied you are at this moment with this area of your life. A dot placed at the center of the circle, close to the middle, indicates dissatisfaction, while a dot placed on the periphery indicates ultimate happiness. Once you have placed a dot in each category, you connect the dots to see your current circle of life. Now you have a clear visual of any imbalances of nourishment, and a starting point for determining where you may wish to spend more time and energy to create balance. Pick the top three areas, circle them and write them down at the bottom of the page. Ask yourself, what's one thing I can do this season to move me in a more joyful direction for this category? Write it down for each category and get started by meditating on the action each day. Ask yourself, "What am I putting off? Why? How am I giving back?

*See the chapter, HOW TO BEGIN, for more explanation of each category

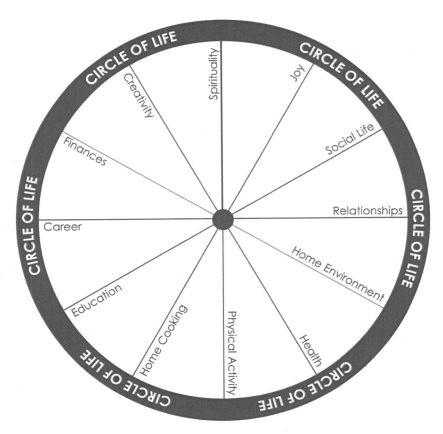

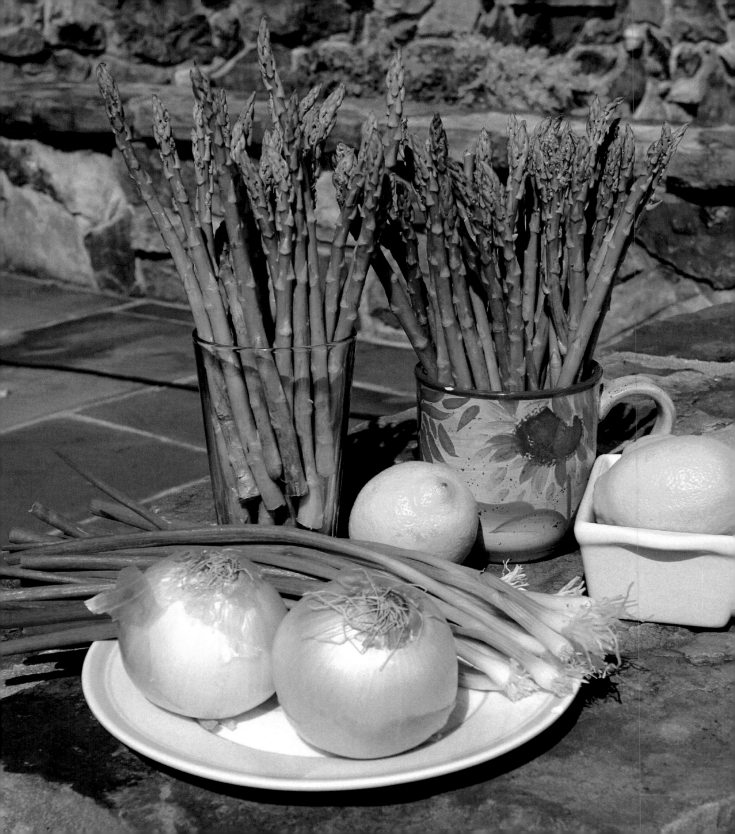

Spring Menus

Lots of cleansing soups this season. Be sure to make extra so you have some for each meal. Beginning each meal with a light soup is a great way to cleanse your system.

MENU 1: Kale & Quinoa Chowder, Whole Grain Bread, Escarole Salad

MENU 2: Miso Soup, Celery Root Salad, Chicken in Parchment with garlic, greens and lemon, Brown Rice

MENU 3: Potassium Broth, Barley & Kale Gratin, Detox Salad

MENU 4: Potato Leek Soup, Poached Fish, Detox Salad

MENU 5: Spring Chicken Soup, Mixed Greens Pizza

MENU 6: Potassium Broth, Crusty Beans & Kale, Onion and Parmesan Pilaf

MENU 7: Miso Soup with Greens, Barley & Spinach Stew, Detox Salad with Sprouts

MENU 8: Potato Leek Soup, Cilantro Citrus Chicken, Gingered Broccoli, Salad

MENU 9: Garlic Broth, Whole Grain Pilaf, White Beans Provençal, Detox Salad

MENU 10: Garlic Broth, Annie's Awesome Salad, Whole Grain Bread

MENU 11: Miso Soup, Chickpea Salad, Mashed Parsnips with Herbs, Detox Salad

MENU 12: Watercress Soup, Spinach & Avocado Salad, Snappy Salmon Burgers or Broiled Salmon with Lemon

ANNIE'S AWESOME SALAD

This is a great salad for a meal. My daughter Sarah (who we call Annie) used to eat this just about everyday. For a vegetarian it fills all the requirements and has a lot of options and flexibility without having to put too much thought into it. Vegans can leave out the eggs and cheese. It's easy to add vegetables based on what is in season while the beans, nuts, seeds, and quinoa give you the protein and complex carbohydrates you need for a balanced plate. I will put aside quinoa and beans from other meals to use in this salad later in the week or for lunch.

Dressing
- 1 lime, freshly squeezed (or lemon)
- 1 teaspoon Dijon mustard
- 1 clove garlic, pressed
- ½ cup yogurt or firm tofu
- ¼ teaspoon sea salt
- ¼ teaspoon freshly ground pepper
- 3 tablespoons extra virgin olive oil

Salad
- 4 cups shredded romaine lettuce, or mixed greens
- 1 cup cherry tomatoes(about 12 small), cut in half, or chopped tomatoes
- 1 cup cucumber, peeled, cored and chopped
- 2 scallions, chopped
- ½ cup orange bell pepper, chopped (optional)
- 1 small yellow squash, or zucchini halved lengthwise and chopped
- 1 small avocado, peeled, cored and chopped
- 1 cup edamame, cooked
- 3 hard-boiled eggs, chopped
- 1 cup baked tofu, chopped into bite-sized pieces (optional)
- ½ cup chickpeas, drained and rinsed, or other bean
- ½ cup quinoa, cooked, or other grain
- 2 tablespoons chives, chopped
- ¼ cup sunflower seeds
- ½ cup fresh herbs like basil, parsley or cilantro, chopped
- Crumbled feta or Gorgonzola cheese, if desired, for topping

▶ Combine the first 6 ingredients in a blender or with a whisk in a small bowl. Gradually add in the olive oil and whisk until well blended. The cheese may be added into the dressing to make a creamy texture or you can sprinkle it over the salad at the end.

▶ Combine the lettuce and the rest of the vegetables in a large bowl. Pour the dressing over the salad and mix well. Add eggs and/or tofu if using and mix again until they are coated. Sprinkle with nuts and/or seeds and chives, fresh herbs, and serve. Top with cheese if you did not include it in the dressing.

Servings: 6

BARLEY & KALE GRATIN

This is a very hearty dish that can serve as a main meal for me. Barley is a great grain to eat in spring as it is very easily digested. It helps to regulate the stomach and fortify the intestines and is high in fiber.

- ⅔ cup barley, rinsed
- Salt and freshly ground pepper
- 1 large bunch kale, rinsed, stems removed and chopped
- 2 tablespoons butter
- 3 tablespoons flour
- 1½ cups veggie stock or milk
- ¼ teaspoon allspice
- ⅛ teaspoon grated nutmeg
- ½ cup Gruyère cheese, or provolone, grated
- 2 cloves garlic, pressed

▶ In a saucepan, add the barley to 1 quart boiling water with ½ teaspoon salt and simmer uncovered until tender, about 30 minutes. Drain.

▶ While the barley is cooking, cook the kale. In a skillet, over medium heat, add the kale and cook for about 3 minutes until kale turns bright green. Add about ½ cup water to the skillet, cover and cook another 5 to 8 minutes stirring to be sure that the kale does not burn. When finished, puree with about ¼ cup of the liquid.

▶ Preheat the oven to 375ºF. Melt the butter in a small saucepan, whisk in the flour and slowly add the broth, making sure to stir constantly in order to prevent lumps from forming. Cook, stirring constantly over medium heat, until thick. Season with spice, nutmeg, salt and pepper. Add pressed garlic. Combine all the ingredients including barley, check the seasonings, then transfer to a lightly buttered baking dish.

▶ Bake until lightly browned on top, about 30 minutes.

Servings: 8 / Yield: ½ cup

BARLEY & SPINACH STEW

This is a nice twist to my normal use of barley. It combines some spicier flavors to perk up the barley and give it some heat. I love topping with the cashews but you could also use walnuts.

- ½ ounce dried mushrooms, sliced
- 3 cups vegetable, chicken or mushroom stock
- ½ cup dry sherry, optional
- 1 tablespoon olive oil
- 1 small onion, finely chopped
- 6 scallions, thinly sliced
- 2 large cloves garlic, crushed
- 1 tablespoon fresh ginger, grated or minced
- 1 teaspoon peppercorns, crushed

- 1 cup barley, rinsed well and drained
- 1 teaspoon sesame oil
- 1 pound baby spinach leaves, slivered
- ⅔ cup cashew nuts, chopped
- 3 tablespoons fresh parsley, chopped
- 1 cup fresh mushrooms like button and shitake, thinly sliced
- Red pepper flakes, optional

▶ Place the mushrooms in a bowl and cover with boiling water, then leave for 15 minutes. Strain, reserving ½ cup of the liquid.

▶ Bring the stock and sherry to a boil in a saucepan, then reduce heat, cover and simmer until needed.

▶ Heat the oil in a large skillet and cook the onions over medium heat for 2 to 3 minutes, or until soft. Add the fresh mushrooms and cook another 3 minutes. Add the garlic, ginger, peppercorns, and scallions and cook for 1 minute. Add the barley and dried mushrooms and mix well. Stir in the mushroom liquid and stock, then reduce the heat and simmer, covered, for about 25 minutes, or until the liquid mostly evaporates. Add more liquid if it evaporates before the 20 minutes are up.

▶ Add the baby spinach to the barley and cover until the spinach wilts, about 1 minute. Mix well. Stir in the parsley, sesame oil and red pepper flakes if using them. Serve topped with the cashews.

Servings: 6

BEET SALAD

My Mom used to make the best beet salad. As a child I didn't like cooked beets warm, but when she added the parsley, garlic, and vinaigrette dressing I could eat the whole bowl. In this version I have also added some Belgian endive and topped it off with goat cheese.

- 6 beets, scrubbed with 1-inch of stem left on the top and all of the root
- 2 Belgian endives sliced crosswise into rounds and separated
- 4 ounces goat cheese

- 2 tablespoons fresh parsley, chopped
- 1 clove garlic, pressed
- 3 tablespoons red wine vinegar
- Sea salt and freshly ground pepper
- Extra virgin olive oil

▶ Steam the beets until they are tender-firm when pierced with a knife, about 25 to 45 minutes depending on the size. Cool, then slip off the skins, and dice.

▶ While the beets are cooking, toss the vinegar, pressed garlic and ¼ teaspoon of sea salt and set aside.

▶ When the beets are ready, toss with the vinegar mixture, taste for salt and season with pepper. Toss with the parsley and endives. Put on individual plates and top with goat cheese. Drizzle your best olive oil over top. Add more pepper, mix everything together and enjoy!

Servings: 6

CHICKPEA SALAD

This is an easy, versatile salad, loaded with protein and great as an accompaniment to any meal. Once made, I often add it to salad greens for lunch.

- 28 ounces chickpeas, cooked or canned
- 4 ounces artichoke hearts, drained and coarsely chopped
- 4 radishes, sliced
- ½ small red onion or scallions, chopped
- ½ cup parsley chopped
- Salt to taste

- Pepper to taste
- 1 clove garlic clove, peeled
- ¼ cup lemon juice, freshly squeezed
- ⅓ cup extra virgin olive oil
- ¼ teaspoon cayenne pepper
- 2 teaspoons cumin powder
- 1 teaspoon fennel seeds, crushed

▶ Combine chickpeas, sliced radishes, chopped artichoke hearts, onions or scallions, and parsley.

▶ Chop and smear the garlic with the side of your knife until it forms a paste. Transfer the paste to a large serving bowl and add the lemon juice.

▶ Stir the spices into the lemon juice. Whisk in the olive oil.

▶ Add the chickpea mixture and toss to combine. Season with salt and serve immediately.

Yields 6 cups

DETOX SALAD

One of my favorite salads for the spring detox time of year. It is so refreshing to eat after a winter of heavier foods. The sprouts are a must! They are high in Vitamin C and offer a high level of vitality. Make sure they are very fresh (be sure to check the date on the package) or grow them yourself. It's very easy. A great base salad for spring cleansing!

- 1 bunch fresh watercress, remove thicker stems
- 2 handfuls arugula
- 1 Belgian endive, chopped
- ¼ pound mushrooms, wiped and sliced
- 1 tablespoon chopped fresh parsley
- 1 green onion, chopped
- Handful of fresh sprouts

Vinaigrette dressing
- Dash of cayenne pepper (optional)
- 1 clove garlic
- 2 teaspoons Dijon style mustard
- ¼ cup freshly squeezed lemon juice
- ¾ cup extra virgin olive oil
- Sea salt and freshly ground pepper

▶ Wash the watercress and tear into bite-sized pieces. Combine the watercress, arugula and endive. Add the mushrooms, green onion and parsley. Keep this mixture in the refrigerator and pull out portions as needed. Add other vegetables.

▶ To make the vinaigrette dressing; mix ¼ cup lemon juice with 2 teaspoons Dijon style mustard, sea salt and pepper to taste, and 1 clove of pressed garlic. Mix well. Add ¾ cups extra virgin olive oil and blend with a whisk or by shaking.

Servings: 5

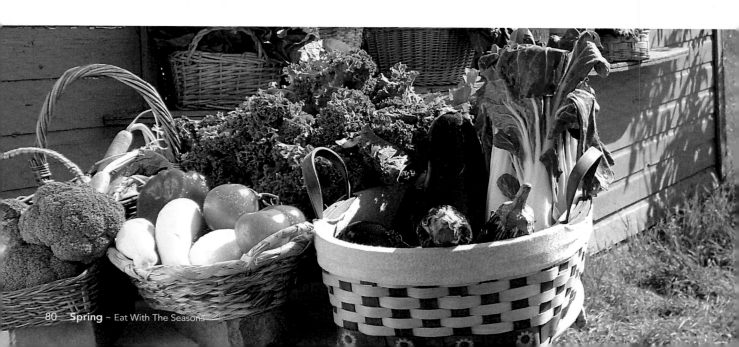

MASHED PARSNIPS WITH HERBS

This is one of my favorite recipes for parsnips. It's so light and the lemon adds just the right amount of zing to the flavor.

- 2 pounds parsnips, peeled and cut into chunks
- ¼ cup plain low fat yogurt
- 2 tablespoons unsalted butter
- 1 tablespoon fresh herbs such as, parsley, chives, dill, mint, chopped
- Finely grated zest of 1 small lemon, and 1 tablespoon lemon juice
- Sea salt and freshly ground pepper to taste

▶ Bring a large pot of salted water to a boil. Add the parsnips and cook until tender when pierced with a fork, 12 to 15 minutes. Drain the parsnips in a colander and let them steam under a clean kitchen towel for about 5 minutes.

▶ Return the parsnips to the pot and mash them with a potato masher, mashing to the consistency you desire. Stir in the yogurt, butter, lemon zest, and juice. Season to taste with salt and pepper. Transfer to a warm serving bowl and sprinkle with herbs and serve.

Servings: 4 / Yield: 6

MISO SOUP WITH GREENS

This is a wonderfully delicious soup for spring. It's nourishing without the heaviness of winter soups. It has leafy greens, mushrooms and seaweed to energize the body and lighten up the diet. Miso is a fermented soybean paste, which is high in protein, trace minerals, and enzymes to give you energy. It comes in different colors depending on what it has been fermented with. The red miso is milder because it is made with white rice. Try the different kinds to decide which you prefer. They all have similar properties.

- 6 cups vegetable stock
- 4-inch piece kombu seaweed
- ¼ cup dried shiitake mushrooms
- 2 cloves garlic
- 2 ounce fresh shiitake mushrooms (stems removed), sliced
- 1 pound leafy greens, like mustard greens, collards, or kale
- 1 tablespoon extra virgin olive oil
- Sea salt to taste
- 1 tablespoon miso
- 1 tablespoon lemon juice
- Freshly ground pepper to taste

▶ In a 4- to 6-quart stockpot, simmer the stock with the kombu and dried mushrooms for 10 minutes. In the meantime, chop the garlic. Wash, trim and chop the greens.

▶ Remove the kombu and mushrooms from the stock. Chop the kombu very finely; set aside. Cut off and discard the stems of both the dried and fresh mushrooms. Slice the caps lengthwise.

▶ In a skillet, heat the oil, add the garlic and sauté for 10 seconds. Add the fresh and dried shiitake, stir, and sprinkle on ¼ teaspoon of the salt. Sauté until the fresh mushrooms wilt, about 4 to 5 minutes.

▶ Add the mushrooms to the stockpot. Swirl a ladleful of stock around the skillet to pick up all the flavors, then return to the stockpot. Add the chopped greens, chopped kombu, and more sea salt to taste if needed. Simmer, uncovered, for 10 to 15 minutes. Adjust the seasoning. Dissolve the miso in the lemon juice and a ladleful of soup stock (if you add it directly to the soup it will clump and have difficulty dissolving). Return to the soup pot. Serve immediately with freshly ground pepper if desired.

Servings: 6

Onion & Parmesan Pilaf

- 2 tablespoons extra virgin olive oil
- 3 medium onions, chopped
- 2 cloves garlic, minced
- 2 cups basmati rice
- 5 cups vegetable stock

- 1½ cups shelled peas
- ½ cup Parmesan cheese freshly grated
- ½ cup fresh parsley leaves, chopped
- ½ cup slivered almonds
- Zest of 1 lemon

▶ In a large pan, heat olive oil, add onion and garlic and stir over low heat for 5 minutes or until soft and golden. Add rice and stock, bring to a boil, stir once. Reduce heat to low; simmer, uncovered, until all the liquid has been absorbed (about 5 minutes).

▶ Add peas, stir until combined. Cover pan, cook over low heat for 10 minutes or until rice is tender. Stir in Parmesan cheese and parsley, serve.

▶ Top with slivered almonds and lemon zest.

Servings: 12

Potato Leek Soup

This is a great soup to eat for dinner after a weekend of over-indulgence. The first time I ever ate this was when I lived in France as a child and my grandmother would often make it as a first course for lunch or dinner. It's heavy enough to complete a light dinner, but light enough for any meal. I will often add watercress at the very end for a variation.

- 1 tablespoon olive oil
- 2 carrots, cut up in larger pieces
- 3 potatoes, cleaned, peeled, cut up
- 1 onion, chopped

- 1 leek, all parts, well cleaned and coarsely chopped
- 3 garlic cloves, peeled and left whole
- 1 quart water, or mix with veggie broth

▶ Put olive oil into a Dutch oven and heat to medium. Add the ingredients, through garlic and sauté for about 3 minutes making sure the oil covers all the vegetables. Add water or broth to cover and bring to a boil. Lower heat to simmer, covered.

▶ Cook for about 20 to 25 minutes until all vegetables are cooked. Add more water or broth if necessary. Use an immersion blender to puree all ingredients or put in a blender. Add salt and pepper to taste and serve.

▶ Top with chopped parsley if desired.

Servings: 6

Quinoa Salad with Asparagus & White Beans

A nice spring salad to take advantage of asparagus when it finally comes back in season.

- 1⅓ cups cooked quinoa
- ½ teaspoon sea salt, to taste
- 1½ tablespoons lemon juice
- 4 tablespoons extra virgin olive oil
- 1 clove garlic, minced or put through a press
- 2 tablespoons basil or mint leaves, chopped
- 1 can (15-ounce) cannellini or great northern beans, drained and rinsed

- ½ pound asparagus, tough ends snapped off, and cut on the bias into 1½-inch pieces
- 1 medium cucumber, chopped finely, peel if skin is bitter
- ½ cup red onion, minced
- Freshly ground black pepper to taste
- Olives (optional)

▶ Bring 1 quart water to boil in medium saucepan. Add asparagus and cook until crisp-tender, about 2 minutes. Drain, rinse asparagus under cold running water, and drain thoroughly again.

▶ In a bowl whisk the lemon juice, pressed garlic, ½ teaspoon of salt, pepper to taste. Add in the olive oil and blend well.

▶ Gently mix the quinoa into the dressing and blend well. Add in the asparagus, cucumbers, beans, onions, and herbs and mix. Eat at room temperature or chill for 30 minutes in an airtight container.

Servings: 4

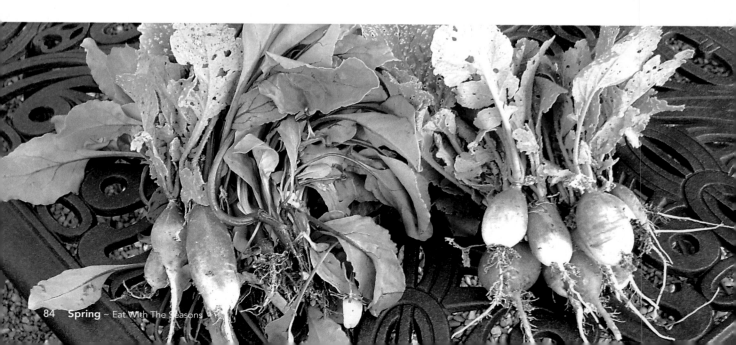

Radish, Celery & Snap Pea Salad

The thing I love about this salad is the crunch. After all the soups and stews of winter, I'm ready for crunching fresh flavors of spring. The bitterness of the radishes and the watery celery are perfect for cleansing the liver.

- 1 bunch radishes, trimmed and thinly sliced
- 1 cup snap peas, trimmed and thinly sliced
- 1 cup celery, thinly sliced, including leaves
- ½ cup scallion, thinly sliced
- ½ cup Romano cheese, shredded
- 1 cup fresh parsley, chopped
- 12 leaves of Boston lettuce

Dressing
- ¼ cup juice from 1 fresh lemon
- 3 tablespoons extra virgin olive oil
- 2 teaspoons whole grain mustard
- ¾ teaspoon sea salt
- 2 cloves garlic, pressed

▶ Whisk the lemon juice, oil, mustard, garlic, and sea salt in a bowl. Add the radishes, snap peas, celery, cheese, parsley; toss to coat. Adjust salt.

▶ Divide the lettuce leaves among 6 plates, top with the salad then garnish with scallions.

Servings: 6

Spinach & Avocado Salad with Warm Mustard Vinaigrette

The healthy fat in avocado gives this salad a very satisfying feeling. The whole grain mustard adds a balancing bitter flavor and a little bite.

- 3 cups baby spinach leaves
- 1 head green leaf lettuce
- 2 medium avocado
- 1 medium cucumber, peeled, seeded and chopped
- 3 tablespoons extra virgin olive oil
- 1 tablespoon sesame seeds, lightly toasted
- 2 tablespoons lemon juice
- 2 teaspoons whole grain mustard
- Sea salt, to taste
- Chopped cilantro, to taste

▶ Wash and thoroughly dry the spinach and lettuce leaves. Tear leaves into bite-size pieces. Place in a large serving bowl.

▶ Cut cucumbers, peel avocados and cut into thin slices. Scatter over the lettuce leaves.

▶ Heat 1 tablespoon of the oil in a small pan. Toast sesame seeds over low heat until lightly browned being careful not to burn. Remove from heat and allow to cool slightly.

▶ Add the lemon juice, remaining oil, and mustard to the pan and whisk to combine. While still warm, pour over the salad and toss gently to coat leaves. Salad is best served immediately.

Servings: 8 / Yield: 8 cups

SPINACH SALAD WITH CRANBERRIES, CROUTONS & GRILLED CHICKEN

Although we think of cranberries in the fall because that is their season, I chose this for spring because of the kidney cleansing properties of cranberries and the soothing digestive qualities of fennel seeds. This is a nice combination of fruit. It can be easily assembled if you have chicken already made ahead. Sometimes I use walnuts instead of pine nuts.

- 1 teaspoon Herbes de Provençe
- ½ teaspoon sea salt
- Chicken breast halves or thighs, skinned and boned (tofu may be used if preferred)
- 4 teaspoons olive oil
- 2 tablespoons shallot, thinly sliced
- 5 garlic cloves, minced
- ¼ cup red wine vinegar
- 1 teaspoon orange rind, grated
- 2 tablespoons pure cranberry juice

- 2 tablespoons honey
- ½ teaspoon fennel seeds, ground in a mortar and pestle
- ½ teaspoon freshly ground black pepper
- ¼ teaspoon kosher salt
- 6 cups baby spinach leaves
- ½ cup dried cranberries
- 2 tablespoons pine nuts, toasted
- 2 tablespoons shallots, thinly sliced
- 2 tablespoons kalamata olive, sliced

▶ To prepare the chicken, combine the Herbes de Provençe with the salt and rub over the chicken. Drizzle olive oil on top and place on a baking sheet and bake for about 30 minutes at 350°F. Or you may cook them in a skillet on the stove in olive oil for about 5 minutes on each side or until done. Remove from the pan and cut into bite size pieces.

▶ To prepare the vinaigrette, add shallots and garlic to pan, cook for 3 minutes or until brown, stirring occasionally. Stir in red wine, orange rind, juice, honey, fennel, pepper and salt; cook over medium high heat until reduced to about ½ cup. Remove from pan and cool.

▶ To prepare the salad, combine spinach, chicken and remaining ingredients in a bowl. Drizzle vinaigrette and toss gently to coat. Serve immediately.

Servings: 6

SPRING CHICKEN SOUP

I learned this recipe from Chef Peter Berley when I took the Master Chef series of classes at Natural Gourmet Institute. I love the lightness of the broth along with the lemon and mint flavors. It's so refreshing yet warming. Sometimes I add a little more rice to make it a little heartier.

- 1- to 3 pound chicken
- 2 quarts water
- 1 cup onion finely chopped
- Sea salt and freshly ground pepper, to taste
- 3 tablespoons medium grain rice like brown or basmati
- ¼ cup freshly squeezed lemon juice
- ½ cup fresh mint, chopped

▶ Combine the chicken and water in a Dutch oven. Bring to a simmer over medium heat. Skim off impurities as they rise to the surface. Add onions and season with salt. Simmer over low heat for 40 minutes to 1 hour. Check on it.

▶ Remove the chicken and transfer the breast meat to a plate. Return the chicken to the pot and simmer 1 hour more. Remove the chicken and cool. Peel away and discard the skin from the chicken and pull the meat from the bones. Slice the reserved breast meat and remaining meat into thin strips and return to the pot.

▶ Add the rice and simmer 15 to 20 minutes until tender. Stir in the lemon juice. Season the soup with salt and pepper.

▶ Place a spoonful of mint in each serving bowl, ladle the soup over it and serve at once.

Servings: 6

WATERCRESS SALAD

A great choice for spring cleansing! I love sardines and they are a great source of omega-3 fatty acids. Since they are at the bottom of the food chain they feed on plankton and do not have the heavy metal contaminants that larger fish have. They are high in calcium and vitamin D and vitamin B12 and have all 8 essential amino acids. I prefer the sardines packed in olive oil. It's best to eat the bones because they are loaded with calcium and are small and soft enough to eat easily.

- 1 bunch fresh watercress, remove thicker stems
- 2 handfuls arugula
- 1 Belgian endive, chopped
- ¼ pound mushrooms, wiped and sliced
- 1 tablespoon chopped fresh parsley
- 1 green onion, chopped
- 1 small can sardines in olive oil (with or without bones)
- Vinaigrette dressing
- Dash of cayenne pepper (optional)

▶ Wash the watercress and tear into bite-sized pieces. Combine the watercress, arugula and endive. Add the mushrooms, green onion and parsley. Lay sardines on top and pour a small amount of vinaigrette over the salad and mix. Top with feta cheese if desired.

▶ To make the vinaigrette dressing; mix ¼ cup lemon juice or red wine vinegar with 2 teaspoons Dijon style mustard, sea salt to taste, and 1 clove of pressed garlic. Mix well. Add ¾ cups extra virgin olive oil and blend with a whisk or by shaking.

Servings: 4

WATERCRESS SOUP

Here is an easy soup very similar to the Potato Leek but with lots of garlic and watercress. Perfect for springtime.

- 1 tablespoon olive oil
- 2 Russet potatoes, peeled and cubed
- 1 onion, chopped
- 2 leek, all parts, cleaned and coarsely chopped
- 2 garlic cloves, peeled and left whole
- 1 quart water, or use veggie broth, or chicken broth
- 1 bunch (or 3 cups) watercress
- Plain low fat yogurt

▶ Put olive oil into a Dutch oven and heat to medium. Add the ingredients, through garlic and sauté for about 3 minutes making sure the oil covers all the vegetables. Add water or broth to cover and bring to a boil. Lower heat to simmer, covered.

▶ Cook for about 20 to 25 minutes until all vegetables are cooked. Add more water or broth if necessary.

▶ Add the watercress and cook for 4 minutes. Use an immersion blender and purée all the ingredients, or put in a blender in batches. Add salt and pepper to taste.

▶ Top with a dollop of plain yogurt, and chopped parsley if desired.

Servings: 6

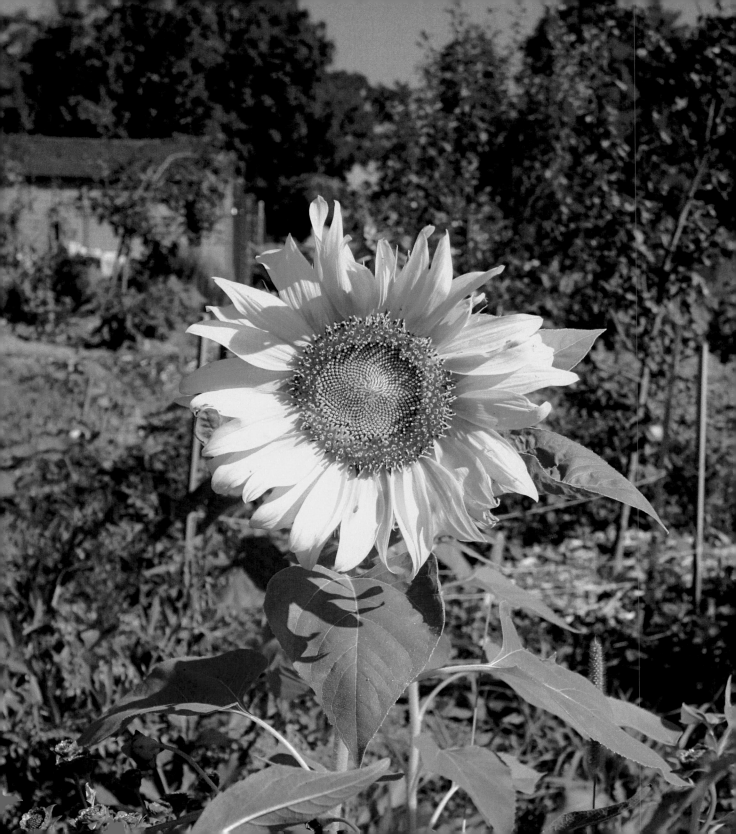

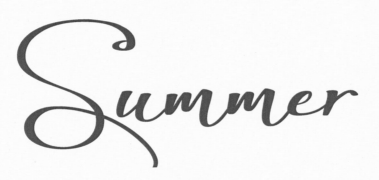

"There is an old Zen saying, 'How you do anything is how you do everything'.
When you rush through meals, you are likely to rush through life."
— DEAN ORNISH

SHIFTING INTO SUMMER

Summer is such an exciting season! The sun is at its most northern position during this season and hits the earth from high above and reflects brightly and makes everything so vivid. Summer Solstice is around June 21 bringing us the longest daylight of the year. This is when the sun reaches its most northern point in the sky at local noon. Nature is bursting with color! The leaves on the trees are a deep green, flowers are blooming everywhere with bright pinks, bold reds, fiery oranges, and vivid yellows. The sun is so warm on my face and I love to soak up the rays and fill my body with all that delicious Vitamin D that I depleted over the winter! The days are nice and long and the rhythm of the season tells me to begin my day with action and mellow into relaxation. There's nothing more enjoyable to me then to sit out on the patio or screen porch on a summer evening listening to the sounds of crickets and frogs, birds and creatures, and feel the warm breeze on my face as I sip a cool beverage.

In the summer there are always so many things to look forward to! All the dreams that blossomed in spring are waiting to be tackled. It's the time to work on projects, get our exercise regime into full swing, tend our gardens, big and small, go on vacations, and relax by the pool or under a shady tree. I always feel so hopeful at the beginning of summer because the days are long and I know that I am going to get so much done!!! From the moment I wake up with the very early sunrise I feel this sense of urgency to get out of bed and get into action! I can hear the birds outside singing and working away at making nests and feeding their babies. All my senses say get going and get outside!! I love to get my exercise done early in the morning when the heat has not quite hit the air. My breakfast is so much lighter with fruit, granola, and yogurt becoming my staples. Berries are so abundant at this time and I love to go from one variety to the next as they come into season. As the summer progresses the farmer's markets abound with colorful vegetables and fruit of the season and the excitement of eating so many delicious and healthy foods. Fresh whole foods taste so delicious with minimal preparation that it's easy to simplify our diet and celebrate the season.

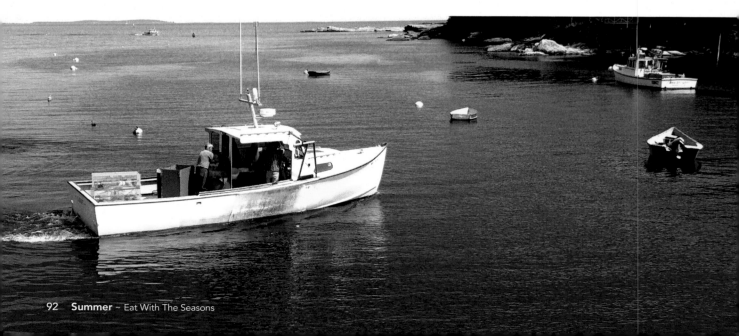

My thoughts on shifting...... KEEP IT LIGHT, FRESH AND SIMPLE.

Summer is the time to really lighten up the diet and eat plenty of fresh, simply prepared whole fruits and vegetables. Think in terms of adding lots of color to your plate so that you eat a variety of foods. Serve salads with cooling foods like sprouts and cucumbers. Eat watery fruits like watermelon. Eat as organic as possible so that you diminish the herbicide and pesticides you ingest but replenish all the minerals and salt that you lose in perspiration. Cook your foods lightly if at all and use high heat for short amounts of time, which makes grilling a perfect method of cooking. Reduce your meat, dairy, and fat consumption so that you feel lighter and don't get sluggish (great time to make bean burgers and bean/grain salads). We often have the urge to drink lots of cold iced drinks and cold foods like ice cream but too much cold can weaken the digestive organs by causing them to contract and stop digestion. Get used to cool beverages or at room temperature if possible. Adding bitter foods to the diet "enters and affects the heart. There it has multiple actions: cleansing the physical heart and associated arteries of deposits;...cooling an overheated heart; and toning up a stagnant liver." (Pitchford pg 338) Eating whole grain salads of wheat or rice which include the germ and bran, with lots of fresh vegetables is a good way to achieve this.

This is also the season to eat some spicy and pungent foods. Adding a little heat to your recipes helps the body to cool down. Add a bit of spice by using fresh ginger root, hot peppers, or black pepper in your diet but do this in moderation so as not to affect your ability to stay warm in cooler weather. Although air conditioning certainly has its place, remember that our body will not adjust to the summer diet unless we get outside as much as possible and help it to feel the shift in temperature and let it adjust (as painful as that might be). If your body still thinks that it's winter it will crave the heavier foods of winter and you might find that you will not lose the weight that can more easily be shed in summer with the lighter diet and the higher activity level. Consider taking morning or evening walks, or doing your summer exercise regime out of doors to bask in the full flavor of summer.

> "Illness can occur when we resist our changes. Illness is usually a process which makes us more receptive, more open to change. This is often its value." Elson Haas M.D.

Summer Seasonal Plan

BREAKFAST OPTIONS: What summer options would you like to add to your breakfast routine? The weather is hot and this is the time of year to eat lots of watery fruits and vegetables. Keep it lighter and cooler but don't neglect your carbohydrates and proteins. Try fresh fruit on whole grain cereal with cool almond or rice milk, or in plain yogurt, crispy raw vegetables, fresh fruit muffins, smoothies are still good. Write down your summer breakfast choices here:

_____

SNACK OPTIONS: This is a great time to snack on fresh fruits and vegetables, hummus with veggies, avocados, homemade frozen yogurt without all the sugar. What are your summer snack choices? Write them here:

_____

LUNCH: What are your all time favorites? Now add in some choices that are seasonal. As the days get very warm you want to keep it cool with salads and clean proteins like fish and chicken, cut up vegetables with herbed sauces and pestos for dipping, veggie sandwiches on sprouted grain bread with lots of sprouts. Write your lunchtime choices here:

_____

MENTAL RECIPE FILE: Go through your mental recipe file and think back to meals you like to make in the summer. Which old stand-by's would you like to keep that are still working for you? Write those here:

_____

NEW SUMMER OPTIONS: Now take a look at the menus in this chapter. Which recipes sound good enough to add to your mental recipe file? Choose 3-4. These are the recipes that you will be working with this summer and making them your own by working with the ingredients to create a meal that is satisfying to your needs. Write the recipe names here:

_____

_____

SUMMER EXERCISE: What changes are you going to make to your summer routine to help you flow with the season? Have you been intending to try a new class, sport, game? Why not put it in your schedule and try it out? This is the time of year to enter that race or challenge that you've always wanted to do. Or learn to play a new sport outside. Take advantage of the longer days while they're here. Write your exercise commitments here:

_____

_____

_____

YOUR SUMMER CIRCLE OF LIFE

Your life at this moment is a direct result of your actions over the last months and years.

This exercise will help you to discover which nourishment you are missing most. The Circle of Life has ten sections. Look at each section of the circle and place a dot on the line to designate how satisfied you are at this moment with this area of your life. A dot placed at the center of the circle, close to the middle, indicates dissatisfaction, while a dot placed on the periphery indicates ultimate happiness. Once you have placed a dot in each category, you connect the dots to see your current circle of life. Now you have a clear visual of any imbalances of nourishment, and a starting point for determining where you may wish to spend more time and energy to create balance. Pick the top three areas, circle them and write them down at the bottom of the page. Ask yourself, what's one thing I can do this season to move me in a more joyful direction for this category? Write it down for each category and get started by meditating on the action each day. Ask yourself, What am I putting off? Why? How am I giving back?

*See the chapter, HOW TO BEGIN, for more explanation of each category.

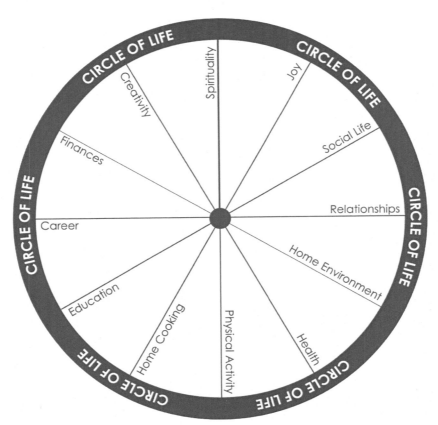

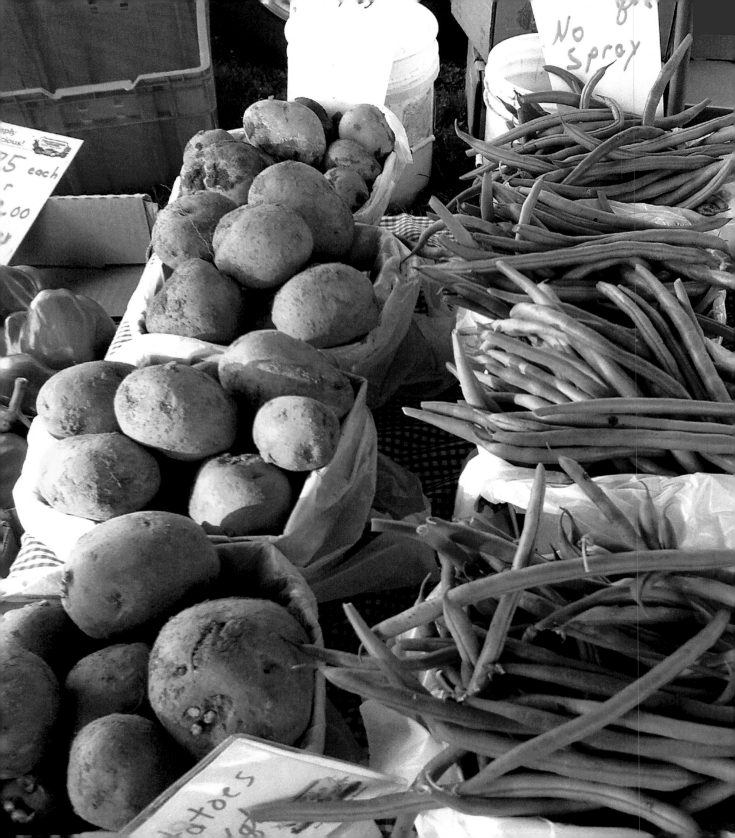

Summer Menus

MENU 1: Soupe au Pistou, Whole Grain Bread, Mixed Greens Salad with Radishes

MENU 2: Sliced Tomatoes with olive oil and sea salt, Quinoa Tabbouleh, Chickpea Salad served over mixed greens

MENU 3: Celery Root Salad, Salade Niçoise with Whole Grain Bread

MENU 4: Cucumbers with lemon/pepper, String bean Salad, Fish/Chicken/Shrimp in Parchment

MENU 5: White Beans a la Provençal, Whole Wheat Couscous, Kale with Feta and Olives

MENU 6: Radishes with sea Salt, Crustless Summer Vegetable Pie made with Swiss chard and spinach, Potato Salad with Celery and Vidalia onions

MENU 7: Sliced tomatoes with extra virgin olive oil, Grilled Marinated Chicken with Blueberry Corn Salsa, Basmati Rice with lemon and parsley

MENU 8: Cucumbers with sea Salt, Summer Tomato Sauce over Udon Noodles topped with Parmesan Cheese, Green Salad with Avocado

MENU 9: String Bean Salad, Black Bean Burgers with Mango Ketchup, Quinoa Tabouleh

MENU 10: Southwest Black Bean Salad with Quinoa, Avocado Toasties

MENU 11: Tomato Salsa with crostinis, Cilantro/Citrus Chicken, Grilled Zucchini

MENU 12: Summer Quinoa Corn Soup, Mediterranean Bean Salad, Pineapple Salsa

Black Bean, Corn & Quinoa Salad

I love this recipe because I can make it seasonal by adding different vegetables. I often leave out the quinoa and use it as a side dish to other grains or burgers.

- ½ cup quinoa, rinsed well and drained
- 1 cup boiling water
- 1 cup kernel corn (from cob or frozen)
- 2 cups black beans, drained and rinsed if using canned
- ¼ cup red onion, chopped
- 1 jalapeño pepper, seeded and finely chopped (optional)
- 2 tomatoes, chopped
- 1 cup cilantro (or parsley), chopped (or to taste)

Mustard Vinaigrette
- 1 clove garlic, minced (or more to taste)
- 3 tablespoons lemon juice, freshly squeezed
- 2 tablespoons lime juice
- 1 tablespoon wine vinegar
- ¼ teaspoon sea salt and pepper to taste
- 2 teaspoons Dijon style mustard
- ¾ cup olive oil

▶ Rinse and drain quinoa. Toast in heated pan. Add water (or stock) and bring to a boil; reduce heat and simmer covered for 15 minutes, until water is absorbed.

▶ After cooking the cobs, remove the corn from each cob and put in a bowl. (If using frozen corn, just defrost and put in bowl.) Add the beans and other ingredients and mix together. Add quinoa after cooling a bit. Add dressing.

▶ For the Vinaigrette Dressing: in a small bowl, combine all ingredients except olive oil. Whisk or shake until well combined. Whisk in olive oil and mix until smooth and well blended (or shake well).

Servings: 6

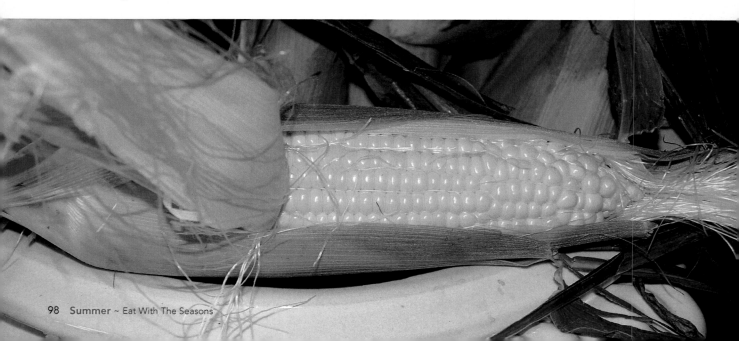

BLUEBERRY CORN SALSA

Every year when we go to Maine I try to get my fill of blueberries (and lobster rolls). It's the season for me to eat blueberry pancakes, blueberry cake and even blueberry ice cream. This recipe combines blueberries with corn for a great summer flavor.

- 4 ears sweet corn kernels
- 4 medium tomatoes, chopped
- 2 small firm avocados, peeled and diced
- 1 small green pepper chopped
- 1 small bunch cilantro, chopped

- 2 limes, juiced
- 2 tablespoons extra virgin olive oil
- 1 tablespoon red wine vinegar
- 2 cups fresh blueberries, rinsed

▶ Cook the corn in boiling water for about 5 minutes, cool, then cut the kernels from the cob.

▶ In a bowl, combine corn with tomatoes, avocados, pepper, cilantro, lime juice, oil, and vinegar until well mixed.

▶ Add the blueberries and mix gently to avoid crushing them. Season with sea salt and freshly ground pepper to taste. Serve over salmon fillets or any other fish or patty you choose.

Servings: 16

CILANTRO CITRUS CHICKEN

Using the easy cilantro-citrus marinade makes for a wonderful, juicy chicken.

- ½ cup chopped onion
- ⅓ cup fresh cilantro leaves
- ¼ cup fresh parsley leaves, chopped
- ¼ cup fresh orange juice
- ¼ cup fresh lime juice
- 2 tablespoons olive oil
- 6 cloves garlic

- 12 skinless, boneless chicken breasts, cut into bite-sized pieces
- 2 teaspoons salt
- 1 teaspoon ground cumin
- ½ teaspoon freshly ground black pepper
- Cooking spray, as needed

▶ Combine first 7 ingredients in a food processor; process until smooth. Place 6 chicken breast halves and half of herb mixture in a large zip-top plastic bag. Place remaining breast halves and remaining herb mixture in a second large zip-top plastic bag, seal and marinate in refrigerator 1 hour, turning bags occasionally.

▶ Prepare grill.

▶ Remove chicken from bag; discard marinade. Let chicken stand 15 minutes. Sprinkle chicken evenly with salt, cumin, and pepper. Place chicken, breast side down, on a grill rack coated with cooking spray. Grill 12 minutes on each side or until a thermometer registers 165°F, turning once.

Servings: 12

CRUST-LESS SUMMER VEGETABLE PIE

This was an old standby in our house. It was easy to put together and get on the table, and I knew all the kids would eat it. Sometimes I add in spinach.

- 8 cups zucchini and/or summer squash, thinly sliced or grated
- 1 cup onions, chopped
- 1 clove garlic, minced
- 2 tablespoons extra virgin olive oil
- 1 large tomato, thinly sliced
- 2 large eggs, beaten
- 1 tablespoon fresh basil, slivered (or parsley)
- 3 ounces goat cheese, crumbled (about ½ cup or so)
- Sea salt and fresh ground pepper

Pistou
- 1 bunch fresh basil
- 2 cloves garlic
- 2 teaspoons extra virgin olive oil

▶ Heat oven to 350°F. Oil 8x8-inch casserole or gratin dish.

▶ Salt zucchini and/or summer squash and let sit in a colander for 15 to 30 minutes. Wipe gently with paper towel and squeeze out the moisture.

▶ To make the pistou, remove leaves from basil stems and place in food processor with garlic and mince. Slowly drizzle olive oil in while blending until mixture is moist but not liquidy.

▶ Heat 1 tablespoon of the oil in a large heavy-bottomed skillet over medium heat and add onions. Sauté until soft. Add squash, salt and pepper. Cook, stirring, for 10 minutes, until the squash is beginning to cook through. Add the garlic and continue to sauté, stirring, for another 5 minutes until the zucchini is fragrant but still bright green. Stir in slivered basil, adjust seasonings and remove from heat. Be sure to drain out any excess liquid.

▶ Beat the eggs together and add the goat cheese, add 1 tablespoon of the pistou (or more to taste), salt and pepper to taste.

▶ Pour zucchini mixture into gratin dish, pour egg mixture over it all, arrange tomato slices on top, crumble 1 tablespoon of goat cheese over the top, drizzle with olive oil.

▶ Bake for 30 minutes, or until eggs are set and top is browned.

Servings: 6

GRILLED PINEAPPLE SALSA

I love pineapples and, although a tropical fruit, I feel they have a place in our diet on a limited basis. Fresh pineapples (not canned or cooked) contain an enzyme called bromelain, which is an anti-inflammatory and a digestive aid. That's why they always serve them at the end of meals in Chinese restaurants. They are also high in Vitamin C and really low in calories. Although we grill the slices in this recipe, it's not enough to kill the enzymes.

- 1 pineapple, cut in rings
- ½ red onion, chopped
- 1 clove garlic, pressed
- ¼ cup cilantro, more to taste, chopped
- 1 tomato, chopped
- 4 tablespoons fresh lemon juice
- ¼ cup extra virgin olive oil
- Salt and pepper to taste

▶ Light the grill and when ready, spray or rub pineapple slices with some olive oil. Place on grill for about 2 minutes on each side and set aside to cool.

▶ In a food processor, put onion, garlic, tomato, lemon juice and pulse just until blended. Add pineapple, olive oil and cilantro and pulse about 3 or 4 times until it is at a consistency that you like.
If you are using it as a ketchup you may want to pulse a little longer than if you are using it as a salsa.

▶ Add salt and pepper to taste and serve.

▶ This is excellent on bean burgers or chickpea patties, or just serve as a salsa with tortillas.

Servings: 8

GRILLED ZUCCHINI WITH LEMON-BALSAMIC VINAIGRETTE

You can really use this topping for any grilled vegetables. It brings a nice thyme / citrus flavor to the vegetables.

- 3 small or medium zucchini (about 1 pound)
- Kosher salt
- 2 tablespoons extra virgin olive oil
- 1 teaspoon extra virgin olive oil
- 1 tablespoon balsamic vinegar
- ½ teaspoon fresh thyme, chopped
- ½ teaspoon lemon zest, finely grated
- Freshly ground black pepper
- 3 tablespoons Parmigiano, freshly grated

▶ Wash the zucchini well to remove any grit and dry them with paper towels. Trim off the ends and slice the zucchini lengthwise into ¼-inch thick slices. Arrange the zucchini on a baking sheet lined with paper towels. Sprinkle with kosher salt and set aside for 10 minutes.

▶ Heat a gas grill to medium high or prepare a medium-hot charcoal fire.

▶ Rub or baste each side of the zucchini with a bit of olive oil. Set the zucchini slices on the grill and cook (if using a gas grill, close the lid), flipping occasionally, until browned and softened but not mushy, 6 to 8 minutes.

▶ Meanwhile, in a small bowl, whisk olive oil, vinegar, thyme, lemon zest, ¼ teaspoon salt, and ⅛ teaspoon pepper.

▶ When the zucchini is grilled, whisk the vinaigrette again and drizzle over the zucchini.

▶ Sprinkle with Parmigiano, adjust the seasonings to taste, and serve immediately.

▶ This can be done with other vegetables like eggplant, onions, peppers. Just adjust the cooking time appropriately.

Servings: 4

GUACAMOLE

I love this recipe. It's simple and the avocados have wonderful essential fatty acids to keep me healthy.

- 3 ripe avocados, preferably Haas
- 1 clove garlic, minced
- 1 lime, juiced
- 1 bunch fresh cilantro, chopped
- Sea salt and pepper, to taste

▶ Peel avocados and remove the pit. In a bowl, or mortar and pestle, mash the avocado with the sea salt until somewhat smooth. (I like to keep chunks in mine because I feel like I get more of the avocado flavor.)

▶ Add in the minced garlic, lime juice, cilantro, and pepper, to taste. Mix and serve.

Servings: 6

KALE WITH FETA & BLACK OLIVES

This easy dish can be made with Swiss Chard too. I love the feta.

- ½ teaspoon kosher salt
- 2 tablespoons olive oil
- ½ small red onion, thinly sliced
- 1 large bunch kale, stemmed and chopped
- 3 cloves garlic, minced
- ¼ cup water
- ½ teaspoon Herbes de Provençe (or a mix of fresh thyme, rosemary, parsley)
- ¼ cup black olives, chopped
- ½ cup feta cheese, crumbled
- Salt and freshly ground pepper, to taste

▶ Heat the olive oil in a large skillet, sauté onions for about 2 minutes or until just tender. Add the kale and garlic, toss to coat with the olive oil. When the kale becomes bright green (after about 2 minutes), add ¼ cup water, and the herbs, cover and cook for about 8 minutes, stirring occasionally and being careful not to let the kale burn. After the kale is cooked, remove the cover.

▶ Stir in the olives and cook a few minutes longer.

▶ Remove from heat, season with salt and pepper to taste, and top with crumbled feta. Serve immediately.

Servings: 4

Mango Ketchup

Not your conventional ketchup from a bottle, this is a great summer blend of fresh tomatoes and mangoes. I love this on bean burgers, fresh veggies and as a dip with tortillas.

- 2 to 3 tomatoes, diced
- 1 mango, peeled and diced
- ½ small red onion, finely diced
- 1 garlic clove, minced
- ¼ cup finely chopped cilantro

- 1½ teaspoon extra virgin olive oil
- 1½ teaspoon fresh lemon juice
- 1 jalapeño pepper, seeded and finely diced,(optional)
- ½ teaspoon sea salt

▶ Place all of the ingredients in a blender and blend until smooth and creamy. Or, blend just enough to keep a salsa texture to it and use as a dip. The ketchup will keep, covered, in the refrigerator for up to 2 weeks.

Servings: 16

Mediterranean Bean Salad

This is a nice summer bean salad that's really easy to make especially if you have lentils on hand.

- 1 can (15-ounce) cannellini beans, rinsed and drained
- ½ cup French lentils, cooked
- ½ cup artichoke hearts, drained and coarsely chopped
- ½ cup zucchini, diced
- ½ cup red onion, diced
- ¼ cup fresh parsley, chopped
- ¼ cup black or green olives, chopped

Dressing
- 3 tablespoons apple cider vinegar
- Juice of 1 lemon
- 6 tablespoons olive oil
- 1 clove garlic, minced
- Sea salt and pepper to taste
- 2 teaspoons Dijon style mustard

▶ In a large bowl, combine beans, lentils, artichokes, onions, zucchini, parsley and olives. Toss with the Dressing.

▶ Cover and let stand for at least 30 minutes or refrigerate overnight. Serve at room temperature.

▶ If using tomatoes, add just before serving.

For Dressing;
▶ In a jar or small bowl, combine oil, vinegar, lemon juice, garlic, mustard, salt and pepper. Shake or whisk to mix well. Taste and add more lemon juice, if desired.

Servings: 4 / Yield: ½ cup

POTATO SALAD

One of my favorite side dishes in summer. I love this version that my mother always made because it doesn't use mayonnaise. If you add the mustard dressing while the potatoes are still warm, it is absorbed into the potatoes and tastes oh so good!

- 2 pounds Yukon Gold potatoes, peeled, cubed
- 2 ribs celery, thinly sliced
- 1 medium onion, chopped
- 1 teaspoon fresh rosemary, minced
- 1 clove garlic, pressed
- Sea salt and freshly ground pepper, to taste
- Mustard vinaigrette (See recipe on page 193.)

▶ Bring a pot of salted water to a boil. Add potatoes and cook until done. You can tell if they're done when a knife inserted into the center comes through easily. Strain water and put into a bowl.

▶ Add dressing, celery, onions, rosemary, and garlic, and mix together well to coat all the potatoes. Let sit for about 30 minutes so the potatoes can absorb the dressing. Season with salt and pepper to taste. You may need to add a little more dressing just before serving.

Servings: 6

Quinoa Tabbouleh

This is a nice light summer salad that doesn't take long to make. While the quinoa cooks you can cut up your vegetables. Add the mint according to your taste buds. I love eating this the next day.

- 1 cup uncooked quinoa, rinsed and drained
- 2 cups water
- ½ teaspoon sea salt and more to taste
- 2 lemons, juiced
- 4 tablespoons extra virgin olive oil
- 2 cloves garlic, minced or put through a press
- ½ cup Italian parsley leaves, chopped
- ½ teaspoon dry mint or mint leaves chopped
- 1 large ripe tomato, chopped
- 1 medium cucumber, chopped finely, peel if skin is bitter
- ½ cup red onion, minced
- Freshly ground black pepper to taste
- Olives (optional)

▶ In a heavy bottomed saucepan bring the quinoa, water and salt to a boil.

▶ Cover and turn to lowest heat. Cook, undisturbed for 15 minutes.

▶ Remove from heat and let quinoa steam for 5 more minutes.

▶ While the quinoa is cooking prepare the other ingredients.

▶ In a bowl combine the rest of the ingredients and season with salt and pepper.

▶ When the quinoa has finished steaming fluff it with a fork.

▶ Transfer the hot quinoa into the bowl.

▶ Gently mix the quinoa into the vegetables. Chill for 30 minutes.

Servings: 6

Tip: For another flavor try making a basil, garlic and olive oil mixture and substitute for the parsley and mint.

SOUPE AU PISTOU

This is a great Provençal recipe for soup that uses fresh basil, garlic and olive oil to add summer flavor. The best part of the soup is when you add the pistou to the bowl and top it with the cheese. I usually add either the vermicelli or the potatoes but not both.

- 1 tablespoon extra virgin olive oil
- 1 medium onion, chopped
- 1 leek, white and light green part, washed and finely sliced
- 1 stick celery, chopped
- 2 medium potatoes, diced
- 2 tomatoes peeled and chopped, or one 8-ounce can of diced tomatoes
- Sea salt, freshly ground pepper
- 8 cups water as needed, or use vegetable or chicken broth
- 8 ounces green beans, cut in short lengths
- ½ cup fresh or cooked navy beans, or other bean of choice
- 2 ounces fine vermicelli, optional

Pistou
- 3 cloves garlic cloves
- 1 bunch basil leaves
- 3 tablespoons olive oil
- 3 tablespoons freshly grated Parmesan or Gruyère cheese

▶ Heat oil in a large saucepan and soften onion and leeks for about 3 minutes. Add celery and potatoes and sauté a few more minutes then add in the tomatoes and garlic and stir.

▶ Add 8 to 10 cups water or stock and salt and pepper. Simmer, covered for about 10 to 15 minutes.

▶ Add green beans, or other veggies like zucchini, beans, and vermicelli and cook 10 minutes more.

▶ Meanwhile, in a food processor, chop garlic finely with basil, gradually adding olive oil and a tablespoon or so of hot liquid from soup. Remove from processor and set aside.

▶ Serve soup in large bowls, spoon in some pistou and sprinkle cheese on top. Use the remainder of the pistou for another dish or freeze in a plastic bag for later use.

Servings: 6

Summer Herb Relish

This relish tastes great with grilled eggplant and any other grilled vegetable. It adds a nice fresh and light taste.

- 2 cups packed fresh parsley leaves
- ½ cup packed fresh mint
- 3 green onions, chopped
- 1½ tablespoon fresh oregano leaves
- 2 tablespoons capers drained
- 3 tablespoons pine nuts
- 1 tablespoon red wine vinegar, or lemon juice
- 2 tablespoons olive oil

▶ Puree ingredients with 5 tablespoons water in blender until smooth.

▶ Season with salt and pepper, if desired.

Servings: 4

Summer Quinoa Corn Soup

This is a great combination of two of my favorite soups with a fresh summer flavor. Serve without the quinoa for a lighter version.

- 6 cups water or stock
- 4 ears organic ears of corn
- 1, 3-inch strip of kombu
- 2 cups cooked quinoa
- 1 tablespoon olive oil
- 1 medium onion, chopped
- 1 stalk celery, chopped
- 2 medium summer squashes, chopped
- 4 teaspoons fresh thyme and marjoram, minced
- 1 teaspoon lemon juice
- Sea salt and freshly ground pepper to taste
- Crumbled feta cheese

▶ In a large pan (big enough for the corn), bring the water or stock to a boil. Add the ears of corn and the kombu and simmer for about 8 minutes. Remove cobs to cool and set liquid aside.

▶ In a large saucepan heat the olive oil over medium heat. Add the onion, and celery and cook, stirring, for about 1 minute. Add the squash, and one teaspoon of the herbs and cook, stirring, until the squash starts to soften.

▶ Add the corn broth, strained of corn silk, rest of the herbs, and salt and bring to a boil. Reduce the heat to a simmer and cook until the squash is soft and translucent, about 5 minutes. (at this point you may use an immersion blender to puree some of the squash to add thickness to your soup).

▶ Meanwhile cut the corn kernels from the ears. When the squash is cooked add the corn to the soup along with the cooked quinoa and the lemon juice.

▶ Serve garnished with feta cheese and more herbs if desired.

Servings: 10

SUMMER TOMATO SAUCE

I love summer tomatoes! They are probably one of my most favorite things to eat, especially right off the vine when they're warm and smell so sunny. We plant several kinds every year and I wait anxiously for them to ripen. We never plant enough for me to freeze because I can't resist eating them fresh. This recipe was invented when my kids were young because I needed to hurry and get dinner on the table. I love to use a really good olive oil, fresh basil, and lots of garlic.

- 2 tablespoons extra virgin olive oil
- 1 to 1½ pounds (4 to 7) ripe tomatoes, chopped
- 1 garlic clove, minced or put through a press
- Salt and freshly ground pepper
- 1 tablespoon slivered basil
- ½ cup grated Parmesan cheese, or more to taste
- ¾ pound whole grain pasta or udon or soba noodles

▶ Heat water for pasta and cook according to directions.

▶ Meanwhile, as pasta is cooking, in a bowl combine tomatoes, olive oil and garlic. Add basil, salt and pepper and toss well. Add grated Parmesan cheese to taste.

▶ Drain noodles, and toss with tomato mixture. Serve with more Parmesan if desired.

Servings: 4

TOMATO BASIL SALSA

Another easy and delicious summer tomato recipe. This has such a great garlicky summer flavor.

- 4 tomatoes, chopped
- 2 cloves garlic, crushed or put through a press
- 2 tablespoons fresh basil, chopped
- 2 tablespoons extra virgin olive oil
- Sea salt and pepper, to taste

▶ Combine all the ingredients in a bowl and mix. Serve as a salsa over grain or bean burgers, as an appetizer with crostini or bruschetta.

Servings: 8 / Yield: 4 cups

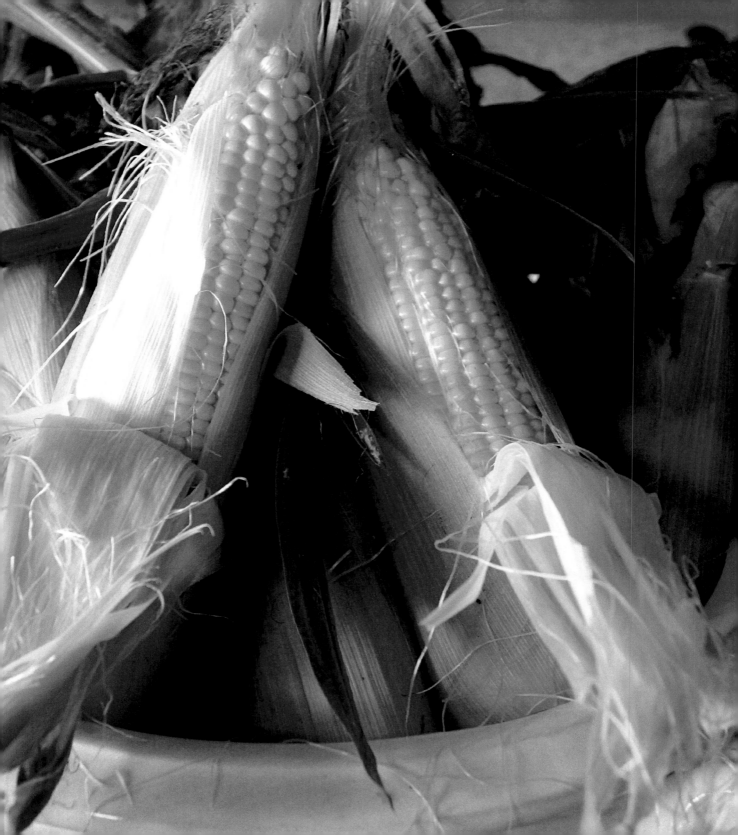

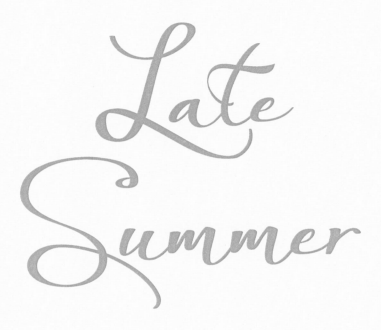

*"Live each season as it passes,
breathe the air, drink the drink,
taste the fruit, and resign yourself
to the influences of each."*
– Henry David Thoreau

SHIFTING INTO LATE SUMMER

In mid-August I always notice a slight shift in how the sun filters through the trees and reflects on the field. It's a little less intense and the leaves are beginning to lose their luscious green as they get ready to show their vibrant fall colors. School buses and children with backpacks begin to reappear, ready for another school year. Autumn is coming! I feel it in the air. Late summer is the time to collect on the earth's bounty and enjoy the fruits of summer's labor. The gardens and markets are loaded with tomatoes, peppers, zucchini, cucumber, eggplant, celery, okra, corn, onions. Peaches are in and apples and squashes are beginning to make an appearance. I love strolling through the vendor stands and feasting on the bounty with my eyes and nose. The scents are like perfume… so earthy and fresh. This is when I love to make my giant sandwich with tons of tomatoes, a good olive oil, some fresh basil, and a wholesome grain bread. So simple yet it speaks volumes to me of warm summer days and time spent in France.

My thoughts on shifting: ENJOY THE WARMTH OF THE SUN ON YOUR FACE AND IN YOUR FOOD

Continue to keep your diet fresh and light as long as summer heat persists. Don't forget to add sprouts to your salads since they are so high in phytonutrients. Eat lots of yellow since corn, yellow peppers, melons are all in season. Continue to keep it simple. The Autumn equinox is September 21 and this is when the darkness will begin to dominate and our balance will begin to shift again. This is a transition time in the year and a good time to manifest the hard work of summer and stay grounded to the earth. As we move from warm weather to cool become aware of the subtle changes in your cravings and, when the urge hits you, begin adding in some roasted vegetables and light soups using the summer harvest foods. These foods will help you to feel more grounded and connected to the earth.

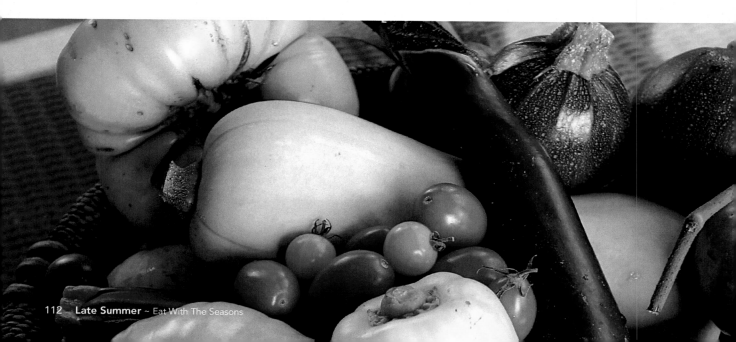

Late Summer Menus

MENU 1: Polenta with Parmesan Cheese, topped with Roasted Tomatoes and Eggplant, White Bean Salad

MENU 2: Quinoa Corn Soup, Giant Summer Sandwich

MENU 3: Healthy Cobb Salad, Whole Grain Bread

MENU 4: Sliced Tomatoes with Olive Oil, Garlic & Basil, Pissaladière, Mediterranean Bean Salad

MENU 5: Saturday Night Special: Autumn Vegetable Pizza (have everyone make their own using roasted summer veggies), Green Salad

MENU 6: Chicken Stew with Olives, Crusty Whole Grain Bread, Green Salad

MENU 7: Ginger Carrot Soup, Mixed Greens Tart, Balsamic Glazed Beets

MENU 8: Vegetable Couscous, Chicken in Parchment or Grilled Marinated Chicken (using lemon, parsley or cilantro)

AUTUMN VEGETABLE PIZZA

This recipe can be made with leftover roasted vegetables of any kind. I am offering a combination of late summer vegetables but you can use tomatoes, eggplant, zucchini just as easily.

Crust
- 1½ cups whole wheat flour
- 1 cup cheddar cheese, grated, or shredded
- ½ cup cornmeal, be sure to use the small granules
- 1 teaspoon sea salt
- 4 tablespoons butter, cut into pieces
- 3 tablespoons extra virgin olive oil
- 3 tablespoons ice water

Pizza
- 2 leeks, white and light green parts only, rinsed and coarsely chopped
- 1 pound broccoli florets, trimmed and cut in half if large

- 1 large fennel bulb, cored and thinly sliced
- 2 medium red onions, chopped into bite-sized pieces
- 1 head garlic
- 2 large beets, peeled and chopped
- 3 large Portobello mushrooms, chopped
- ½ teaspoon sea salt
- Freshly ground pepper to taste
- 1 tablespoon Herbes de Provençe, or other favorite herb mix
- 2 tablespoons extra virgin olive oil
- ⅓ cup Tapenade*
- ½ cup goat cheese, crumbled

▶ Prepare either a 9x13-inch casserole dish or a large pizza pan or quiche dish by spraying the bottom with olive oil. In the food processor, place the flour, cheddar cheese, salt, and cornmeal; pulse to combine. Add the butter, one piece at a time, pulsing after each addition until blended. Add oil and water and pulse until the dough begins to come together. Turn the dough into your prepared pan of choice, spread the dough evenly and press firmly into the bottom and up the sides of the pan to make your pizza crust. Refrigerate until you are ready to bake.

To Roast the Vegetables;

▶ Place cut up vegetables in a baggie or in a bowl. Add olive oil, Herbes de Provençe (or any other herb blend that you like), seal the bag and be sure the air is out. Massage the vegetables so that the oil and herbs cover all the vegetables. Pour onto a baking sheet covered with parchment paper, making sure to spread the vegetables out in one thick layer. Bake in the oven at 375° for about 30 minutes or until veggies are tender, stirring once half way through.

▶ When all the veggies are done, remove from oven and reduce the oven to 350°F. Bake the crust until it is set but not browned, about 15 minutes.

▶ Remove crust from the oven and let cool for a few minutes. Spread the tapenade over the bottom of the crust. Top with the roasted veggies. Squeeze the garlic out of the cloves and onto the vegetables. Top with the crumbled goat cheese. You can top with olives if desired.

▶ Bake in the oven until the edges are brown, about 25 minutes. Let it cool for about 10 minutes before cutting or removing from the pan.

Servings: 8   *For Tapenade recipe see page 192 or, purchase pre-made at the store.*

BALSAMIC GLAZED BEETS

One of my favorite ways to make beets. When I'm craving iron I can eat these warm beets right out of the pan and I feel better right away. Beets are high in antioxidant phytonutrients and have been shown to protect the liver from free radicals which could lead to cancerous activity. Their nutrients are great for energy, bone strength, and heart health. Eating the greens adds to their antioxidant potential.

- 1 medium red onion
- 1 bunch fresh beets with tops
- 3 tablespoons balsamic vinegar
- 2 tablespoons extra virgin olive oil
- 2 sprigs fresh tarragon, leaves finely chopped
- ½ teaspoon sea salt, or to taste
- Freshly ground pepper

▶ Peel the onion and halve it lengthwise. Cut each half into ¼-inch thick crescents from root to stem and set aside.

▶ Cut the tops off the beets, leaving 1 inch of stems attached to each beet. Trim the root ends and scrub the beets with a stiff brush to remove any grit.

▶ Cut each beet into 4 to 6 wedges, depending on their size. Wash the greens and stems in several changes of cold water. Drain, coarsely chop, and set aside.

▶ In a heavy pan wide enough to hold the vegetables in a snug single layer, combine the onions, beets, vinegar, butter or oil, tarragon, and salt. Pour enough water to barely cover the vegetables and bring to a boil over high heat. Reduce the heat to low, and simmer, covered, for 25 minutes or until the beets are nearly, but not quite tender.

▶ Raise the heat and boil, uncovered, until the liquid has reduces to a syrup and the beets are fork-tender.

▶ Add the beet greens, reduce the heat, and simmer, covered, for 5 minutes. Uncover the pan and turn the greens over so they mix with the beets and onions. Add the black pepper and additional salt to taste. Simmer 2 minutes longer and serve.

Servings: 8

CHICKEN STEW WITH OLIVES

This comes from a version of a recipe that I learned when I went to the South of France and took a wonderful Market to Table cooking class with Rosa Jackson at Les Petits Farcis. We walked through the market in Nice, visited lots of vendors and stalls and had delicious samplings of everything from wine to olive oil. After we bought our fresh chicken from the vendor we went back to her place and made a similar recipe with lots of garlic and olives.

- 1 frying chicken, cut into pieces
- Sea salt and freshly ground pepper
- Chickpea flour
- ¼ cup extra virgin olive oil
- 1 small onion, finely chopped
- 1 leek, chopped
- ½ cup dry white wine
- 1 pound fresh, chopped, organic tomatoes (or 28-ounce can diced tomatoes)
- 3 medium zucchini, chopped
- 1 green pepper, chopped (optional)
- 4 cloves garlic, minced
- 1 bunch parsley
- ⅔ cups black olives
- Fresh basil leaves

▶ Season the chicken pieces with salt and pepper, then coat with chickpea flour, shaking off excess.

▶ In a large sauté pan over medium heat, warm olive oil. Put chicken pieces in the pan except for breasts. Sauté, turning the pieces for 10 minutes. Add the breast and sauté until all pieces are nicely colored on both sides, about 10 minutes longer. Reduce heat to low, cover and simmer for 10 minutes.

▶ Transfer chicken to a warmed platter. Keep warm. Add onion and leeks to the pan and stir around with a wooden spoon. When it begins to color, pour in the wine. Raise the heat to high and deglaze the pan, scraping the pan bottom with a wooden spoon until the brown bits dissolve and the wine is almost completely reduced. Add the tomatoes, zucchini and pepper and salt to taste and continue to cook over high heat, shaking the pan and stirring, until their excess liquid evaporates. Add the chicken pieces and stir together. A couple of minutes before removing from the heat, add parsley/garlic mixture and olives. Top with basil leaves. Serve.

Servings: 6

GINGER-CARROT SOUP

This is a simple soup with a powerful punch. Ginger has strong anti-inflammatory properties as well as the ability to soothe the stomach and nausea. Its fresh flavor gives a zip to any dish. Try adding it to other dishes for its health and flavor properties.

- 2 tablespoons olive oil
- 2 medium onions, chopped
- 2 pounds carrots peeled and diced
- 2 sweet potatoes, peeled and cubed, or use a butternut squash cut into pieces.
- 1, 2-inch ginger root, peeled and minced
- 28 ounces chicken or veggie broth
- Salt and freshly ground black pepper to taste

▶ Sauté first 5 ingredients for about 5 minutes. Add just enough liquid to cover the vegetables plus about another 1½-inches, and simmer until vegetables are cooked through.

▶ When the soup is cooked, use an immersion blender (or put in the blender) and puree until smooth.

▶ Serve warm. Add a dollop of crème fraiche, yogurt or cream, for added richness.

Servings: 4

Healthy Cobb Salad

A great alternative to a typical Cobb salad that has all the bacon and heavy dressing. I like this lighter version with eggs but sometimes I add chicken also.

Dressing
- Juice from 1 lime, freshly squeezed
- 1 teaspoon Dijon mustard
- 1 clove garlic, pressed
- ½ cup yogurt or firm tofu
- ¼ teaspoon sea salt
- ¼ teaspoon freshly ground pepper
- 3 tablespoons extra virgin olive oil

Salad
- 1 cup cherry tomatoes (about 12 small), cut in half
- 1 cup cucumber, peeled, cored and chopped
- ½ cup radishes, sliced
- 2 scallions, chopped
- ½ cup orange bell pepper, optional, chopped
- 1 Small yellow squash, halved lengthwise and sliced
- 1 small avocado, peeled, cored and chopped
- 4 cups shredded romaine lettuce
- 2 tablespoons chives, chopped
- ¼ cup almonds, toasted
- Crumbled Gorgonzola cheese, if desired, for topping
- 3 hard-boiled eggs, chopped or grilled chicken, chopped, or baked tofu, chopped

▶ Combine the first 6 ingredients in a blender or with a whisk in a small bowl. Gradually add in the olive oil and whisk until well blended. The Gorgonzola cheese may be added into the dressing to make a creamy texture or you can sprinkle it over the salad at the end.

▶ Combine the next 7 ingredients, (if using peppers), and the lettuce, in a large bowl. Pour the dressing over the salad and mix well. Add eggs or chicken or tofu if using and mix again until they are coated. Add in eggs and/or chicken if using. Sprinkle with almonds and chives and serve. Top with Gorgonzola cheese if you did not include it in the dressing.

Servings: 6

MIXED GREENS TART

I like this recipe in my repertoire because it helps to get the all-important leafy greens into my diet, it's a complete meal, and the leftovers taste great for lunch the next day. I feel like I can get a lot of mileage out of it. It's especially easy if I've cooked some greens and rice for a meal earlier in the week. Set some aside for this quick dish.

- 2 pounds Swiss chard, kale, beet greens, or any mix of greens such as spinach, collards, arugula, bok choy, stems removed and chopped into ribbons
- 2 tablespoons olive oil
- 1 large onion, chopped
- 2 to 4 cloves garlic, minced or put through a press
- 2 bunches of parsley, chopped
- ½ cup short grain brown rice (optional)
- 2 tablespoons chopped fresh rosemary or 1 tablespoon crushed dried (optional)
- 1 to 2 teaspoons fresh thyme leaves or ½ teaspoon dried
- 2 ounces Gruyère cheese, grated (½ cup)
- 2 tablespoons freshly grated Paremsan cheese
- 3 large eggs, beaten
- 1 tart crust, half-baked

▶ Wash the greens well. Heat 1 tablespoon olive oil in a large skillet over medium heat and add the wet greens, putting the tougher greens in first. Cook, stirring, until they wilt in the water left on their leaves, about 8 minutes. Remove from the heat and transfer to a colander. Allow to cool, then squeeze dry. Set aside.

▶ Preheat the oven to 400°F. Heat the rest of the olive oil in the same skillet over medium-low heat and add the onions. Cook, stirring, until the onion begins to soften, about 3 minutes. Add the garlic. Stir in the greens, parsley, herbs, salt and pepper (and optional rice). Transfer to a bowl and stir in the cheeses and eggs. Adjust the seasonings and turn into the crust.

▶ Bake until eggs are set, about 35 to 45 minutes. Allow to rest before serving. Can be served cold.

Servings: 8

Pissaladière - Onion Tart

This pizza type snack is great as a starter for a light meal, or it can be the meal if you add a nice green salad and maybe a soup before. It's absolutely one of my favorite things to eat. The traditional French version has olives and anchovies only, but I like to add some goat cheese to the top.

- 3 tablespoon olive oil (or more as needed)
- 4 to 5 good-sized onions, very thinly sliced
- 1 sprig of thyme (¼ teaspoon dried)
- 1 bay leaf
- 3 garlic cloves, crushed
- Sea salt and freshly ground pepper
- 6 to 12 anchovy fillets in oil, drained
- About 15 Niçoise type olives (cured)

Recipe for pizza dough or Savory Pastry Dough
- 1 tablespoon dry yeast
- ¼ cup warm water
- 1½ cups flour, unbleached and unbromated*
- 1 teaspoon sea salt
- 1 teaspoon sugar
- 2 tablespoons extra virgin olive oil
- 1 egg, at room temperature

▶ In a small bowl, dissolve the yeast in the water. In a mixing bowl, combine the flour, salt and sugar. Make a well in the center and add the olive oil, egg, and yeast water mixture. Using one hand, combine to form a dough, then turn out the dough and knead for at least 5 minutes (you can also make the dough in a food processor or a mixer with a dough hook.)

▶ **For the topping;** Heat olive oil in a large skillet. Add the onions, cover and sauté them in olive oil over low heat until translucent but not browned, about 10 minutes, stirring from time to time to prevent browning.

▶ After about 10 minutes, add thyme, bay leaf. Keep the heat low and let onions caramelize, stirring periodically until they turn golden brown, without sticking to the pan.

▶ After another 15 minutes lift the lid and add the garlic. Season with salt and extra pepper. Add water if necessary to prevent them from sticking. Remove cover, stir and continue cooking, checking periodically, for a total of about 45 minutes.

▶ Preheat the oven to 475°F. Roll out the dough, place on a baking sheet and spread the onion mixture on top. Arrange the anchovy fillets on top and dot with the olives. Sprinkle with a little olive oil and bake for 30 minutes.

▶ Serve hot, warm, or at room temperature. If you like, scatter a little more thyme before serving.

Servings: 4

Unbromated means that it has not been treated with potassium bromate, a chemical oxidizer that may be toxic to the endocrine glands and is possibly carcinogenic to humans according to the International Agency for Research on Cancer.

POLENTA WITH ONION & THYME

With the sweet taste of onions and the fresh thyme, this version of polenta adds to the feel of late summer.
Put a topping on this or eat plain as a side dish.

- 5 cups water, plus additional boiling water in a kettle
- 1 teaspoon salt
- 1⅓ cups coarse stone-ground cornmeal
- 2 tablespoons extra virgin olive oil
- 1 onion, finely diced
- 2 tablespoons fresh thyme leaves

▶ Bring the water to a boil in a deep heavy pot. Have additional water in a kettle. Add the salt and reduce the heat so the water is just boiling — a little higher than a simmer. Using a long handled wooden spoon, stir the water constantly in one direction while you add the cornmeal in a very slow stream, so slow that you can see the individual grains. The mixture will become harder and harder to stir as you add all the cornmeal. If it seems extremely thick, add boiling water from the kettle, a little at a time.

▶ Once all the cornmeal has been added, continue to stir the same direction for about 20 minutes. The polenta should come away from the sides of the pan when it's done. It may seem that it's done before 20 minutes but continue to add more water as the polenta will not have the creamy consistency if stopped too soon. The spoon should be able to stand up in the middle.

▶ In the meantime, heat the olive oil in a sauté pan. Add the onions and sauté until browned, about 8 minutes. Stir into the polenta as it cooks.

▶ Stir in the thyme and salt to taste.

▶ Pour polenta onto a lightly oiled cookie sheet or baking pan and cool until firm, about ½ hour. Cut into squares and sauté, bake, grill, or broil.

Servings: 4

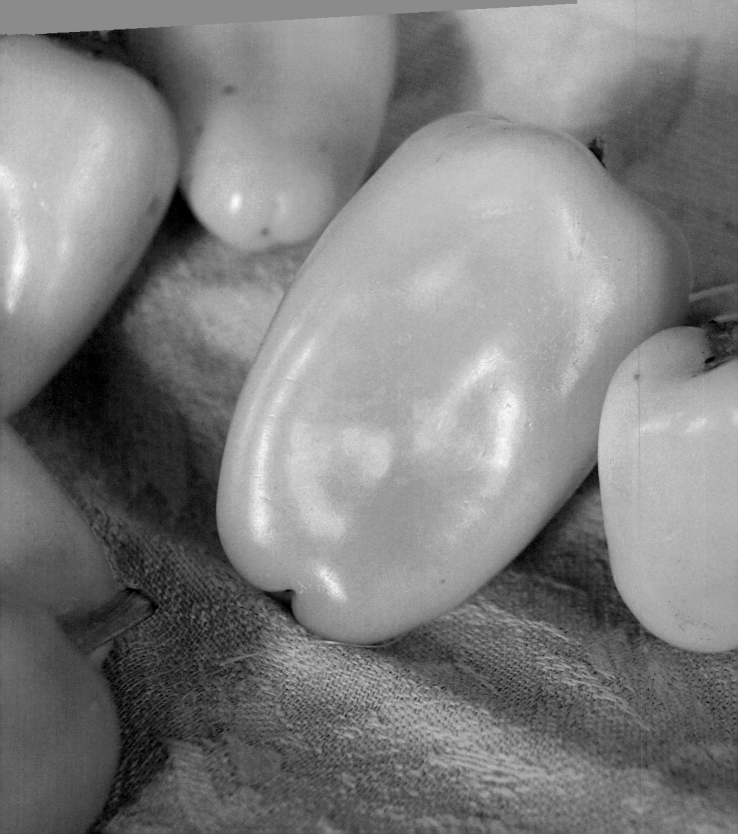

RATATOUILLE

This recipe exemplifies all the flavors of the Late Summer season. The garden basket is brimming with "nightshade" vegetables which include tomatoes, peppers, and eggplant, and this recipe mixes them together for a warm smokey, end of summer flavor.

- 1 large eggplant, peeled and sliced lengthwise
- 2 onions, sliced
- 4 cloves garlic, sliced
- 2 zucchini, cut lengthwise and sliced ½-inch thick
- 2 red or green peppers, seeded and sliced
- 1 pound tomatoes, canned or fresh, peeled (if using fresh), and diced
- 3 to 4 tablespoons extra virgin olive oil
- 1 bay leaf
- 1 teaspoon fresh thyme
- 1 tablespoon fresh basil, chopped
- Sea salt and freshly ground pepper, to taste

▶ Heat the oven to 350°F. Oil a baking sheet (or you can use parchment paper) and place eggplant, inside down, on the baking sheet and bake for about 20 minutes or until soft. Prepare the other vegetables while baking.

▶ Heat oil over medium-low heat in a heavy-bottomed casserole or sauté pan and gently sauté onions and garlic until onion is tender. Add the peppers and sauté for a few minutes. Add zucchini and sauté just a few minutes until soft.

▶ Add tomatoes and herbs, stir together, then place mixture in a casserole.

▶ Remove the eggplant from the oven and let cool a few minutes, then dice. Add to the casserole and mix everything together.

▶ Put the casserole in the oven and bake, covered for 30 minutes. Remove the cover and bake another 20 minutes.

▶ Add salt to taste and plenty of freshly ground pepper. You may also want to add more herbs or a bit of cayenne pepper.

▶ Serve hot or cold. Top with Parmesan cheese, or goat or feta cheese. Serve with polenta, rice or couscous.

Servings: 8

ROASTED TOMATOES & EGGPLANT
WITH BASIL & GARLIC

This is a great do-ahead recipe. You can roast the vegetables ahead and have them ready for stacking onto grilled polenta, burgers, or just plain in a sandwich. Be sure to make extra for eating right out of the oven. The tomatoes taste so sweet they don't last long in my house!

- 4 small, Italian eggplants, sliced lengthwise into ¼-inch pieces
- 4 ripe tomatoes, sliced
- 2 tablespoons extra virgin olive oil

Pistou
- 1 clove garlic
- 1 bunch fresh basil, about ½ cup
- 1 tablespoon extra virgin olive oil, or so

▶ Preheat oven to 375°F.

▶ Place eggplant slices on a baking sheet, brush with olive oil and bake for about 20 minutes until done.

▶ Slice tomatoes about ¼-inch thick, drizzle with olive oil and bake on parchment for about 30 minutes, or until they have lost their juices and look sturdy. These two steps can be done simultaneously.

For the Pistou;

▶ Put the basil, garlic and sea salt in a food processor and mix. Add olive oil until it becomes a paste.

▶ After removing vegetables from the oven, brush with the basil garlic mixture. Make a stack from the vegetables, drizzle with more olive oil, sea salt and pepper and serve.

Servings: 8

SPICY RED LENTIL SOUP

Don't let the long list of ingredients fool you. This is a 3-step recipe that just involves adding all the herbs and spices to the pot. This recipe gets a spicy kick from harissa, a hot Moroccan condiment made by preserving chile peppers in oil and salt. Top the soup with plain yogurt to cool it off.

- 1½ teaspoon virgin olive oil
- ½ cup chopped onion
- 1 teaspoon minced garlic
- 1½ teaspoon minced peeled fresh ginger
- ¾ teaspoon paprika
- ½ teaspoon sea salt
- ¼ teaspoon ground cumin
- ⅛ teaspoon freshly ground pepper

- 3 cups stock (chicken or veggie)
- 1 cup dried red lentils, rinsed and drained
- 1 cup canned chickpeas, rinsed and drained
- 1 can (14-ounce) diced tomatoes, undrained
- 1 tablespoon fresh lemon juice
- 1 teaspoon harissa (see page 188) (or chile powder or other spicy powder)
- Chopped fresh cilantro (optional)

▶ Heat oil in a large saucepan over medium heat. Add onion and garlic and cook until tender, stirring frequently. Stir in ginger, paprika, salt, cumin, and pepper and cook 1 minute.

▶ Add 3 cups stock, lentils, chickpeas and tomatoes and bring to a boil.

▶ Cover, reduce heat, and simmer for 30 minutes or until the lentils are tender, stirring occasionally. Puree some of the soup if you prefer to have a thick soup. Stir in lemon juice and harissa.

▶ Garnish with fresh, chopped cilantro if desired.

Servings: 6

THE GIANT SUMMER SANDWICH

This sandwich is inspired from the Provençal Pan Bagnat, which combines the fresh flavors of warm summer in a sandwich with a delicious vinaigrette. It's a big seller in the South of France and tastes so delicious when eating it outside in the warm sun. My daughter and I shared one of these eating experiences sitting on a bench overlooking the blue azure of the Mediterranean and enjoying every messy bite we ate. This is the time to use your favorite extra virgin olive oil to drizzle. Be sure to have plenty of napkins. I eat mine with anchovies and it adds the finishing touch!

- 1 large, (1 pound) loaf ciabatta or other round country style loaf

Herb Vinaigrette
- ¼ cup fresh basil leaves
- 1 tablespoon fresh marjoram, chopped
- 1 tablespoon fresh parsley leaves, chopped
- 1 small garlic clove, minced
- 4 teaspoons red wine vinegar
- 2 teaspoons Dijon style mustard
- Sea salt and freshly ground pepper to taste
- ⅓ cup extra virgin olive oil

Sandwich
- 2 or more large ripe tomatoes, sliced
- 1 large yellow or red bell pepper, roasted, peeled and quartered
- 4 ounces goat, fresh mozzarella, or other favorite cheese, sliced
- Sea salt and freshly ground pepper to taste
- 8 to 9 black olives, like Kalamata or niçoise
- Several anchovies for topping (optional)

▶ For the vinaigrette; In a small bowl, finely chop the herbs with the garlic. Add the mustard, salt and pepper, and vinegar and blend well with a whisk. Add the olive oil and mix until well blended. Adjust seasonings if needed.

▶ Slice the top third of the loaf of bread and set it aside. Pull out the inside (and use later to make breadcrumbs).

▶ Spread the inside with some of the dressing, then make layers of the sliced tomatoes, pepper, cheese, olives. Top with anchovies if using. Drizzle a bit of your favorite extra virgin olive oil over the top.

▶ Add the top of the bread, press down, then cut into large pieces.

▶ If you use a mini-loaf you can keep it all to yourself!

Servings: 4

VEGETABLE COUSCOUS

This is a nice meal that can also be served over quinoa or rice. The vegetables can change with the seasons but I especially like to eat this in late summer on to fall and winter.

- 1½ teaspoon virgin olive oil
- ½ cup chopped onion
- 1 teaspoon minced garlic
- 1½ teaspoon minced peeled fresh ginger
- ¾ teaspoon paprika
- ½ teaspoon sea salt
- ¼ teaspoon ground cumin
- ⅛ teaspoon freshly ground pepper
- 3 cups stock (chicken or veggie)
- 1 cup dried red lentils, rinsed and drained
- 1 cup of canned chickpeas, rinsed and drained
- 1 can (14-ounce) diced tomatoes, undrained
- 1 cup whole wheat couscous
- 1 tablespoon fresh lemon juice
- 1 teaspoon harissa (see page 188)
  (or chile powder or other spicy powder)
- Chopped fresh cilantro and parsely (optional)

▶ Heat the olive oil in a large heavy-bottomed soup pot. Add the onion, half the garlic, and the green pepper, sauté until the onion begins to soften.

▶ Add the leeks, celery, canned tomatoes, water or stock, and bay leaf. Cook for 10 minutes.

▶ Add saffron, remaining garlic, carrots, squash and other vegetables (except zucchini), salt and pepper to taste, cover and simmer 15 minutes.

▶ Add zucchini and cayenne pepper to taste and adjust seasonings. Cook for 5 more minutes.

Set aside and prepare couscous:

▶ Bring 1½ cups water or stock to a boil with a teaspoon of olive oil.

▶ Add the couscous, stir and cover and let sit for about 5 minutes. When ready to serve, fluff with a fork.

▶ Spoon couscous into soup bowls and ladle a generous serving of the soup. Garnish with lemon, harissa (be sure to dissolve in broth first), cilantro and parsley.

Servings: 8

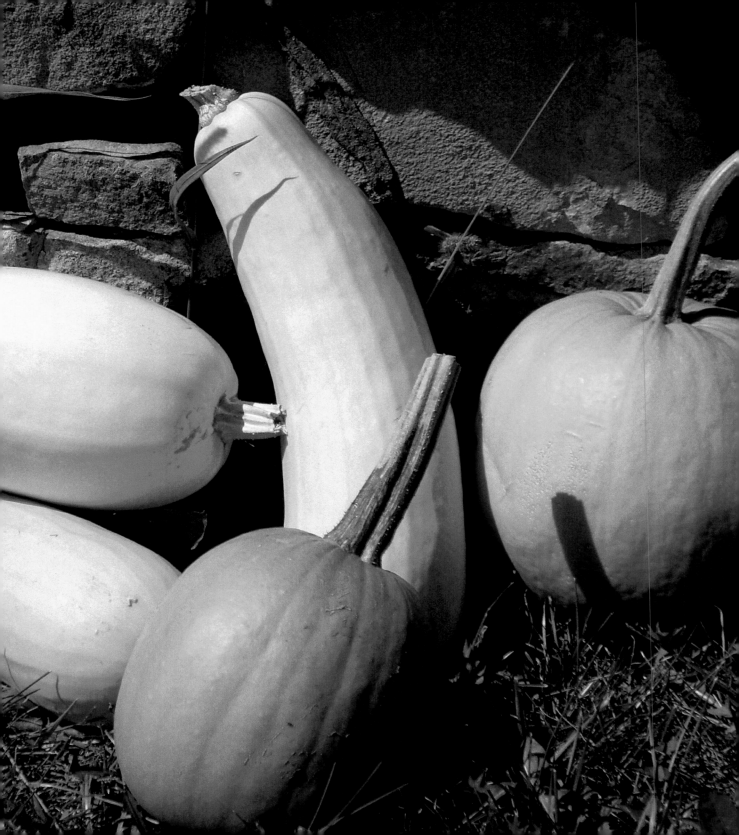

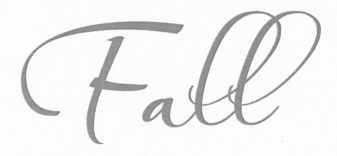

"Take care of your body with steadfast fidelity. The soul must see through these eyes alone, and if they are dim, the whole world is clouded."
— Johann Wolfgang von Goethe

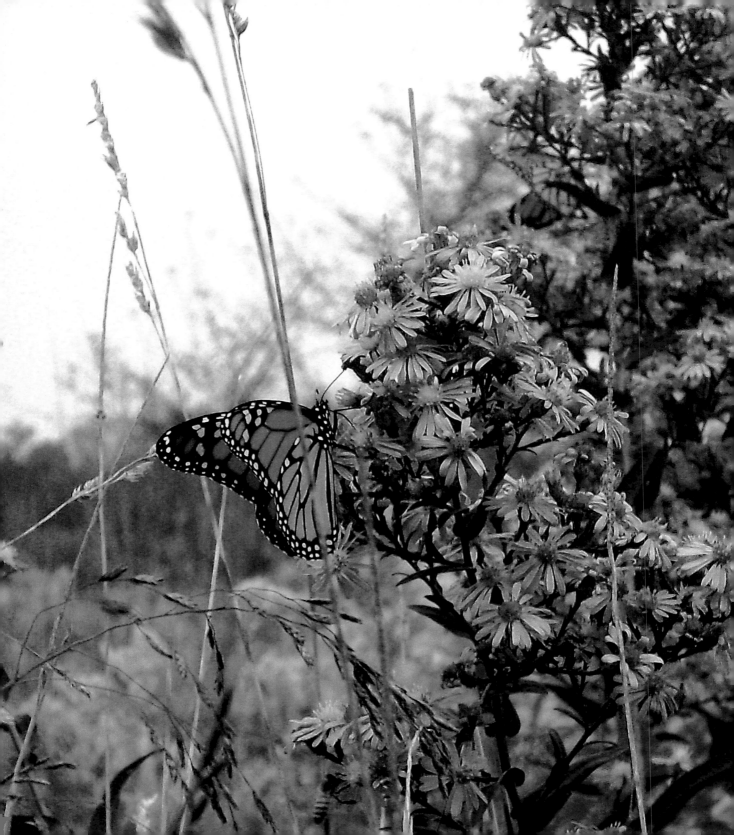

SHIFTING INTO FALL

I love early morning in the fall when everything is still. The ribbons of mist rise up from the streams and low-lying fields and my home on the hill has a story book feel. The dew sparkles on the grass as the rising sun casts its golden light onto the fading yellow goldenrod and the browning tall grasses. The pastures are vibrant green waiting for the first frost to arrive. I see the cows on the neighbor's farm meandering slowly, searching for their last green energy food before winter sets in and they must survive on hay. I notice that I feel the same way...craving a last blast of green energizing foods before I shift into eating heartier soups and more cooked vegetables and desserts, all in an effort to prepare my body for winter. I love the beautiful squashes and pumpkins that are sprawled all over the garden waiting to be picked. The kale is growing, waiting for the first frost to make it sweeter. The root vegetables like parsnips, beets, carrots, turnips, are all ready to give me the grounding, warm energy I will need this winter.

My thoughts on shifting: CELEBRATE THE HARVEST

The Autumnal equinox occurs in mid-September. This is when the sun crosses the equator. If spring and summer are the seasons of expending great energy, autumn is now the time to gather all our energy to store for winter's rest period. Just as the harvest is plentiful and we celebrate Thanksgiving with a hearty meal, so we are preparing our bodies for a season of moving inward for the darker days of winter. I always feel like a busy beaver doing yard work, winterizing the garden, putting in the winter crop bulbs like garlic and daffodils, raking leaves, and finishing up the outside projects where the work was too hot to do in summer. If you have a history of catching colds then it's time to take care to nourish yourself. The air can be very dry in the fall and the blowing wind makes it easy to get chilled. The windy weather often makes me feel scattered and flighty. It's important to be sure you get enough water and eat foods that moisten the body like, millet, barley, spinach, persimmon, honey, sesame seeds, rice syrup, almonds, pears, apples and, this is a good time to eat soy products like tofu and tempeh. This is also the time to nourish the lungs and large intestines. An imbalance in these areas can often be associated with increased mucus, runny nose, sinus congestion, coughs and colds. This is the time to begin eating foods that are pungent and spicy in order to open the senses and clear the sinuses to stimulate the lungs. They aid in assimilation and the absorption of food. Add more foods like; sour apples, lemons, apple cider vinegar, yogurt, sauerkraut, pickles, leeks, hot peppers, along with spices like black pepper, ginger root, fennel seeds, turmeric. A good snack for fall would be a spicy trail mix. I start to look forward to making soups, roasted root vegetables and squashes right about this time. Baking and sautéeing concentrated foods can help to thicken the blood and keep the body warm. I add in the longer roasting proteins like beef stews, (from grass fed beef) and chicken soup with lots of carrots and celery. I usually increase my cooked vegetables and fruit to 80 percent with fresh salads to top off my meal.

> "Viruses cannot attack a healthy human organism. Prevention and cure for the common cold is to stay in tune with your life." – Elson Haas

FALL SEASONAL PLAN

BREAKFAST OPTIONS: What fall options would you like to add to your breakfast routine? Apples and pears are in season now. Heartier porridge, like oats or buckwheat, with almond milk and raisins and cinnamon can be very warming and satisfying. Write down your fall breakfast choices here:

_____

SNACK OPTIONS: Add in dried fruit, nuts and seeds to your snack choices along with fresh apples and pears. Try roasting pumpkin seeds for a quick healthy snack. Add in a hint of spicy herbs like cayenne pepper. What are your fall snack choices? Write them here:

_____

LUNCH: What are your all time favorites? Now add in some choices that are seasonal. As the days get cooler you might want to bring along warming soups, salads that have more than lettuce in them like the wheat berry-cranberry salad, and seasonal roasted vegetables. Write your lunchtime choices here:

_____

MENTAL RECIPE FILE: Go through your mental recipe file and think back to meals you like to make in the fall. Which old stand-by's would you like to keep that are satisfying and still working for you? Write those here:

_____

NEW FALL OPTIONS: Now take a look at the menus in this chapter. Which recipes sound good enough to add to your mental recipe file? Choose 3 to 4. These are the recipes that you will be working with this fall and making them your own by working with the ingredients to create a meal that is satisfying to your needs. Write the recipe names here:

_____

_____

FALL EXERCISE: What changes are you going to make to your fall routine to help you flow with the season? Have you been intending to try a new class, sport, game? Why not put it in your schedule and try it out? This is a great season for joining a local race as a runner or walker. There are so many good causes to walk/run for and give back! Write your exercise commitments here:

_____

_____

_____

YOUR FALL CIRCLE OF LIFE

Your life at this moment is a direct result of your actions over the last months and years.

This exercise will help you to discover which nourishing foods you are missing most. The Circle of Life has ten sections. Look at each section of the circle and place a dot on the line to designate how satisfied you are at this moment with this area of your life. A dot placed at the center of the circle, close to the middle, indicate dissatisfaction, while a dot placed on the periphery indicates ultimate happiness. Once you have placed a dot in each category, you connect the dots to see your current circle of life. Now you have a clear visual of any imbalances of nourishing foods, and a starting point for determining where you may wish to spend more time and energy to create balance. Pick the top three areas, circle them and write them down at the bottom of the page. Ask yourself, what's one thing I can do this season to move me in a more joyful direction for this category? Write it down for each category and get started by meditating on the action each day. Ask yourself, What am I putting off? Why? How am I giving back?

*See the chapter, HOW TO BEGIN, for more explanation of each category.

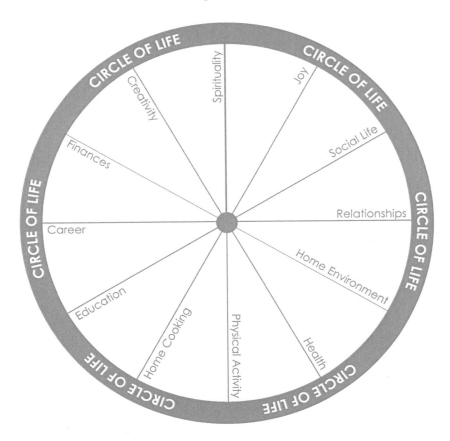

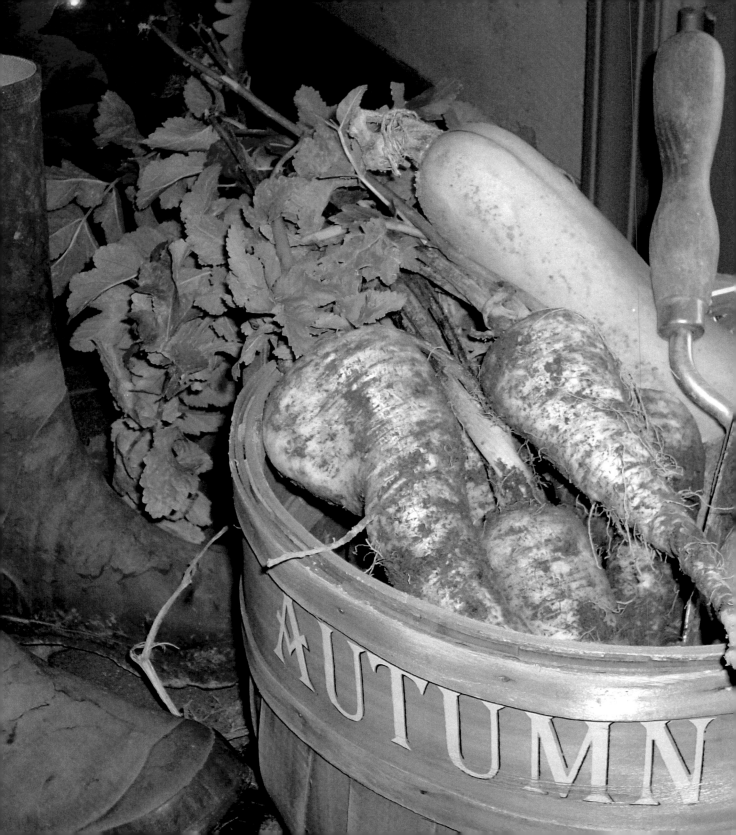

FALL MENUS

MENU 1: Leafy Greens Shepherd's Pie (make extra kale) with Roasted Chicken (make 2 and use one for leftovers), Apple, Walnut, Endive Salad(without the quinoa) eaten at the end of the meal

MENU 2: Stuffed Delicata Squash with Chard or Kale (from day before), Quinoa & White Beans. (make extra quinoa to use later in the week), Green Salad

MENU 3: Easy Quinoa Bake, Roasted Squash with Garlic & Parsley, Gingered Broccoli

MENU 4: Harvest Squash Soup or Roasted Squash Soup, Turkey Meatloaf, Brussels Sprouts with Cauliflower

MENU 5: Chickpea Patties with Herbed Tofu/Yogurt Spread, Sweet Carrots, Cilantro-Lime Rice, Green Salad

MENU 6: Polenta Pizza with Vegetables of Choice, Apple, Walnut & Endive Salad (with or without quinoa)

MENU 7: Vegetable Bulgur Chili with toppings of choice, Cilantro-Lime Rice, Green Salad

MENU 8: Miso Soup, Baked Portobello Mushrooms with Millet, Gingered Broccoli topped with Sesame Seeds

MENU 9: French Lentils, Butternut Squash Gratin over whole wheat couscous, Green Salad with Escarole

MENU 10: Greek Bison Burgers, Cider Roasted Root Vegetables or Peppery Parsnip Fries, Mixed Leafy Greens sautéed in extra virgin olive oil

MENU 11: Easy Dinner Omelet with Spinach/Kale, Balsamic Glazed Beets, Escarole Salad

MENU 12: Millet & Sweet Potato Patties with Herbed Yogurt, Easy Cabbage, Green Escarole Salad with Mustard Vinaigrette

MENU 13: Chicken Stew Provençal, Whole Grain Bread, Salad

APPLE, WALNUT & ENDIVE SALAD

I like this salad in the winter because of the mix of nuts, apples and watery Belgian Endive. Sometimes I leave the quinoa out altogether if I'm eating it as a side dish.

- 1 cup apples, diced
- 2 cups arugula
- 1 cup Belgian endive, pulled apart and sliced
- ¼ cup walnuts, crushed
- ½ cup water or broth
- ¼ cup quinoa, rinsed well and drained
- 3 tablespoons fresh lemon juice

Dressing
- 1 cup plain, low fat yogurt
- 4 tablespoons goat cheese, or to taste
- 2 tablespoons apple cider vinegar
- 1 tablespoon fresh parsley, or other herbs to taste, minced
- ¼ teaspoon garlic powder, or 1 clove pressed garlic
- Sea salt and freshly ground pepper to taste

▶ **To cook the quinoa;** after draining the quinoa, place in a saucepan or high skillet and toast over medium high heat, for about 4 minutes. Add the water or broth to the toasted quinoa and bring to a boil. Reduce heat to a simmer and cook for about 10 minutes, or until done. The water will be absorbed. Remove from the heat and set aside to cool. (This step can be done ahead of time in conjunction with another meal and you can just set some aside for this salad.)

▶ In a bowl, combine the apples, quinoa, walnuts and drizzle with lemon juice.

▶ On a salad platter, arrange the arugula, top with the endive leaves, and put the apple mixture over top.

▶ Drizzle with the Goat Cheese Dressing or your favorite vinaigrette. Mix well and serve.

▶ Dressing; Makes about 1 cup. Mix all the ingredients in a blender or with a whisk. Add salt and pepper to taste and drizzle over salad. (You could also make the dressing without the goat cheese and then just crumble some goat cheese over the salad.)

▶ Alternate Dressing: ½ cup walnut oil (or ¼ cup olive oil and ¼ cup walnut oil), ¼ cup apple cider vinegar, crisp apple, peeled, cored and chopped, ¼ teaspoon garlic powder, pinch paprika, sea salt and freshly ground pepper, to taste. Puree all ingredients in a blender or food processor.

Asian Coleslaw

The thing I like about this coleslaw is that it has a nice spicy flavor that pairs well with recipes that are a little more simple in taste. I like to serve it with grain recipes and bean recipes, or even alongside an omelet to give me a zesty, crunchy flavor. It adds the spicy flavor that is needed in the fall to clear the sinuses and stimulate the lungs. Cabbage is high in Vitamin C and other nutrients, high in fiber, and rich in sulfur nutrients to help fight infections. Eating in the cruciferous family of vegetables is a great way to prepare for the winter virus season.

- 2 cups red cabbage, shredded
- 2 cups Napa cabbage, shredded
- 2 large carrots, grated
- 1 small red onion, minced
- 1 jalapeño chile pepper, seeded and minced
- 1 medium apple, thinly sliced
- 1 tablespoons toasted sesame oil
- 4 tablespoons extra virgin olive oil
- 5 tablespoons rice vinegar
- 1 tablespoon agave nectar
- ½ teaspoon Asian chile garlic sauce, or more to taste
- 1 tablespoon fresh ginger root, peeled and finely grated
- Sea salt, to taste
- ½ cup almonds, slivered
- 4 tablespoons toasted sesame seeds, or a sesame seed blend

▶ Place the red cabbage, Napa cabbage, carrots, onions and jalapeño in a large bowl. Stir to combine.

▶ Place the sesame oil, olive oil, vinegar, chile sauce, agave nectar, and ginger in a glass jar and seal the lid tightly. Shake the jar vigorously to combine (or whisk in a bowl). Taste for seasoning, adding more salt or chile garlic if needed. Pour the dressing over the cabbage mixture and toss to combine. Refrigerate, covered, for 2 to 4 hours to allow flavors to blend.

▶ When ready to serve, remove coleslaw from the refrigerator, add the apples and almonds to the salad and toss again, adding more dressing if needed. Top with sesame seeds and serve.

Servings: 6

BAKED PORTOBELLO MUSHROOMS STUFFED WITH HERBED MILLET

I love millet for its alkalizing properties. It also strengthens the kidneys, is high in protein, rich in silicon (for joint strength), high in B Vitamins, calcium, iron, magnesium, and potassium, and is gluten-free. People who have celiac disease or are gluten intolerant are better able to digest millet because it does not contain any gluten. I sometimes make this recipe for millet without using it as a stuffing. It makes a great side dish.

- ⅓ cup oil-packed sun-dried tomatoes, drained and finely chopped
- 2 tablespoons oil from the jar
- 4 green onions, thinly sliced
- 2 cloves garlic, minced
- 1 teaspoon fresh rosemary, finely chopped
- 1 cup millet
- 3 cups water or broth
- ½ cup grated Parmesan cheese, divided
- 4 medium portobello mushroom caps
- 1 tomato, sliced

For the millet;

▶ Heat 1 tablespoon of the sun-dried tomato oil in a saucepan over medium heat. Add the sun-dried tomatoes, green onions, garlic and rosemary, and cook for 5 minutes, or until onions are soft, stirring constantly. Add the millet, and cook 1 minute.

▶ Add 3 cups water or broth (or a mix), cover and reduce heat to medium low. Simmer 25 to 30 minutes, or until millet is tender and all water has been absorbed. Remove from the heat and stir in ¼ cup cheese. Season with salt and pepper to taste.

For the mushrooms;

▶ Preheat the oven to 400°F. Coat a baking sheet with olive oil. Scrape the gills from the mushroom caps. Brush with remaining oil from tomatoes, season with Herbes de Provençe if desired, place cap side up on the baking sheet. Divide the millet mixture among the mushroom caps, mounding slightly to fill. Sprinkle with remaining cheese, and top with a tomato slice. Bake 20 to 25 minutes, or until browned and cheese has melted.

Servings: 4

BRUSSELS SPROUTS WITH CAULIFLOWER & A MUSTARD-CAPER BUTTER

I had not been a big fan of Brussels Sprouts in the past until my sister started to bring them to our Thanksgiving table. They were so very delicious that I looked for other ways to prepare them. They have all the cancer-fighting properties of cabbage and are a great addition to the diet. I thought I would include this recipe along with the cauliflower because they come in season around the same time. The caper sauce adds a nice touch.

- 1 pound Brussels sprouts
- 1 small head of white cauliflower
- 1 small head of broccoli or other cauliflower colors
- Sea salt and freshly ground pepper, to taste

Mustard-Caper Butter
- 2 cloves garlic
- 6 tablespoons unsalted butter at room temperature
- 2 teaspoons Dijon style mustard
- ¼ cup small capers, drained and rinsed
- 1 lemon, zested
- 3 tablespoons marjoram, chopped

▶ Pound the garlic with ½ teaspoon salt in a mortar until smooth, then stir it into the butter with the mustard, capers, lemon zest, and marjoram. The butter can be made a day ahead and refrigerated. Bring to room temperature before serving.

▶ Trim the base off the sprouts, then slice them in half or, if large, into quarters. Cut the cauliflower and broccoli into bite-sized pieces.

▶ Bring a large pot of water to a boil and add salt. Add the Brussels sprouts and cook for 3 minutes. Then add the other vegetables and continue to cook until tender, about 5 minutes. Drain, shake off any excess water, then toss with the Mustard-Caper Butter. Taste for salt, season with pepper and toss again. Serve immediately.

Tip: You can also cut all the vegetables into bite-sized pieces, mix with the mustard butter and roast in 350°F oven for about 20 to 30 minutes.

Servings: 8

BUTTERNUT SQUASH GRATIN WITH GRUYÈRE & SAGE

Butternut is my favorite winter squash. It's a little lighter and tastes great in soups, gratin, baked, or puréed. It blends very well with Gruyère cheese in this recipe.

- 4 teaspoons olive oil
- 2 cups onion, thinly sliced
- 1 tablespoon fresh sage, chopped
- 4 sprigs thyme
- Sea salt and fresh ground pepper
- 5 cups butternut squash peeled and cut into 1-inch cubes
- ½ cup flour
- 2 tablespoons fresh parsley, chopped
- ½ cup stock (chicken or veggie)
- ½ cup Gruyère cheese, grated, or Gorgonzola cheese, crumbled
- 2 tablespoons breadcrumbs, (natural brand without additives like Panko)

▶ Preheat the oven to 350°F. Lightly oil a 2-quart gratin dish.

▶ Heat half the oil in a skillet over medium heat. Add the onion, thyme, and sage and cook, stirring frequently, until the onions are lightly caramelized, about 10 minutes. Season with ½ teaspoon sea salt and pepper to taste. Spread in the gratin dish, return the skillet to medium heat and add the remaining oil. Toss the squash in the flour, letting the excess fall away. Add it to the pan and cook until it begins to brown in places on both sides, about 7 minutes. Add the parsley, season with salt and pepper, and cook for 1 minute more. Layer the squash mixture over the onions and mix gently. Add ½ cup or stock.

▶ Cover the squash and bake for 20 minutes, or until squash is tender.

▶ Remove from oven, sprinkle with cheese and breadcrumbs and bake an additional 10 minutes until cheese is melted and crumbs are golden brown.

Servings: 6

CIDER-GLAZED ROOTS
WITH CINNAMON WALNUTS

This is a nice twist to roasted root vegetables that can also take care of a sweet tooth in a nutritious way.
Makes a great side dish for the Holiday Table.

- 3 pounds assorted root vegetables, such as carrots, parsnips, sweet potatoes, beets, peeled and cut into 1-inch pieces
- 1 cup apple cider
- ¼ cup maple syrup
- ½ teaspoon sea salt
- ¼ teaspoon fresh ground pepper
- 1 tablespoon butter
- ⅛ teaspoon ground cinnamon
- 1 cup walnuts, roughly chopped

▶ Preheat oven to 400°F.

▶ If using parsnips, quarter lengthwise and remove the woody core from the bigger stalks before cutting into 1-inch pieces. Whisk cider, maple syrup, ½ teaspoon salt, and pepper in a 9x13-inch baking dish. Add root vegetables and toss to coat. Cover the baking dish with foil.

▶ Bake for 20 minutes. Uncover and stir the vegetables. Continue cooking, uncovered, stirring every 20 minutes or so, until the vegetables are glazed and tender, about 1 hour or more.

▶ Meanwhile, place walnuts in a small skillet and cook over medium-high heat, stirring constantly, until fragrant and lightly browned, 2 to 6 minutes. Remove from the heat and add butter, cinnamon and a pinch of salt. Stir until butter is melted and the nuts are coated. Spread out on a plate to cool slightly.

▶ Transfer the vegetables to a serving dish and sprinkle with the cinnamon walnuts.

Servings: 6

Delicata Squash Stuffed
with Chard, Quinoa & White Beans

I included this recipe because it's delicious, but it also makes a great vegetarian holiday meal to accompany the turkey eaters. A bit labor intensive but you can make most of it ahead of time and then assemble the day of.

- 2 medium squashes such as Delicata or Acorn, halved and seeded
- 1 teaspoon plus 2 tablespoons virgin olive oil
- 6 cloves garlic, unpeeled
- ½ teaspoon sea salt
- ½ teaspoon ground pepper
- ½ cup onion, chopped
- 1 clove garlic, minced
- 2 tablespoons water or broth
- 1 tablespoon tomato paste

- 1 sprig thyme leaves
- ¼ teaspoon sage leaves, chopped
- 8 cups chard leaves or kale, chopped in ribbons
- 1½ cups white beans, or one 15-ounce can, rinsed
- ¼ cup Kalamata olives, chopped
- 2 cups cooked quinoa
- ⅓ cup breadcrumbs
- ¼ cup Parmesan cheese, freshly grated
- ½ cup Gruyère cheese, grated

▶ Heat oven to 350°F. After cutting and seeding the squash, brush the insides with olive oil, sprinkle with salt and pepper, and place face down on the baking sheet with 3 garlic cloves inside each half. Bake for about 30 minutes, or until tender. When finished baking, remove garlic, take off skin, mash in a bowl, and save to add to the chard mixture.

▶ Meanwhile, heat 1 tablespoon olive oil in a large skillet over medium heat. Add onion; cook, stirring until starting to brown, 2 to 3 minutes. Add minced garlic and stir for one more minute. Stir in water, tomato paste, herbs, and sprinkle with salt and pepper. Stir in the chard, cover and cook until tender, about 6 minutes. Stir in the white beans, mashed roasted garlic, quinoa and olives; cook until heated through, about 1 or 2 more minutes.

▶ Position rack in the center of the oven and preheat the broiler.

▶ Combine the breadcrumbs, Parmesan and about 1 tablespoon olive oil in a bowl. Fill each squash half with about 1 cup of the chard mixture. Place in a baking sheet (slicing the bottom of each squash if necessary, to make it stay balanced). Sprinkle the breadcrumb mixture on top of each. Top with Gruyère cheese and broil until lightly browned, about 1 to 2 minutes.

Servings: 4

EASY CABBAGE

Cabbage is so abundant and inexpensive in the fall. It is just one of the cruciferous vegetables that are high in sulfur compounds which aid the liver in producing enzymes to detoxify. It's a great source of Vitamin C which is an antioxidant that helps protect the cells from disease and helps in the fight against tumors. There are many kinds of cabbage like; green, red, savoy, bok choy, napa. This recipe is an easy way to sauté and bring out the sweetness. It tastes better each day you cook it so make lots.

- 1 head green or red cabbage, chopped
- 1 large onion, chopped
- 2 cloves garlic clove, minced
- ½ cup water
- 2 tablespoons olive oil

- Apple cider vinegar or umeboshi or plum vinegar for finishing
- 2 teaspoons dried thyme, or Herbes de Provençe blend, (if using fresh thyme then use 1 tablespoon)

▶ Put chopped cabbage in a skillet with water, cover and let cook for about 5 minutes on high.

▶ Remove cover, discard any excess water, add olive oil and onions and sauté for another 5 minutes.

▶ Add the garlic, stir and cook for 3 minutes. Serve topped with salt and pepper, vinegar of choice, and any other condiment you may enjoy.

Servings: 6

French Lentils

Although this looks like a long recipe, it's an easy one-pot meal. Lentils are known to be beneficial to the heart and to stimulate circulation. A great addition to the diet.

- ½ pound French green lentils, rinsed
- ¼ cup extra virgin olive oil
- 2 cups yellow onions, chopped
- 2 cups leeks, white and light green parts only, rinsed and coarsely chopped
- 1 teaspoon thyme leaves
- 2 teaspoons kosher salt

- ¾ teaspoon freshly ground black pepper
- 1 tablespoon fresh garlic minced
- 1½ cups celery, chopped (4 stalks)
- 1½ cups carrots, chopped (3 carrots)
- 1½ cups water, vegetable or chicken broth
- 2 tablespoons tomato paste
- 2 tablespoons red wine vinegar

▶ Place lentils in a heat-proof bowl and cover with boiling water. Set aside for 15 minutes, then drain.

▶ Meanwhile, heat the oil in a sauté pan, add the onions, leeks, thyme, salt, and pepper and cook over medium heat for 10 minutes, until the onions are translucent. Add the garlic and cook for 2 more minutes. Add the celery, carrots, lentils, stock or water, and tomato paste. Cover and simmer over low heat for 20 minutes, until the lentils are tender.

▶ Add the vinegar and season to taste.

Servings: 6

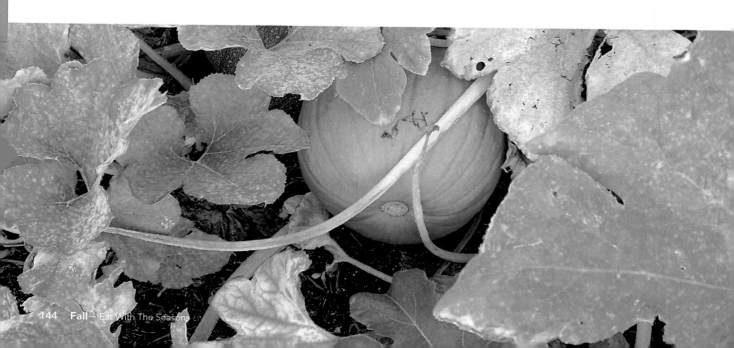

GARLIC GINGERED BROCCOLI
WITH TOASTED PUMPKIN SEEDS

This is one of my favorite ways to prepare broccoli. The ginger root and garlic mix so well together to enhance the broccoli flavor. The added tamari adds a little zip, and the pumpkin seeds a little crunch.

- 1 bunch broccoli
- 3 cloves garlic, minced
- 3-inch piece fresh ginger, finely grated or minced
- 6 cups water

- 1 tablespoon olive oil
- 2 tablespoons tamari soy sauce
- Toasted pumpkin seeds, (see recipe page 43)

▶ Wash and cut broccoli into florets. You can use the stems, but it will take longer to cook.

▶ Add 6 cups water to a pot. Bring to boil.

▶ Drop in your broccoli and let quick boil for about 3 minutes. Remove from water and give them a quick rinse.

▶ Heat olive oil in skillet over medium-high heat. Add garlic and sauté for a few seconds (be careful not to burn garlic). Add broccoli and sauté for several minutes until bright green and just tender. Add tamari soy sauce and ginger. Toss. Top with toasted pumpkin seeds.

Servings: 4

CELERY ROOT SALAD

This is one of my all time favorite salads. It reminds me of France because that is the first place I ever tasted it. It was very common for my grandmother to make as a first course for dinner. Celery root is high in silicon which is great for connective tissue and bone strength. I also make this same salad with carrots and add parsley to it. So delicious either way.

- 1 celery root, peeled and grated

Vinaigrette dressing

- ¼ cup apple cider vinegar
- 2 tablespoons Dijon mustard

- ¾ cup olive oil
- 1 garlic clove, pressed
- Sea salt, ground pepper

▶ Grate celery root into bowl. Combine ingredients for vinaigrette dressing and add pressed garlic and mix. Pour over celery root and mix well. Season with sea salt and fresh ground pepper as desired. Serve at room temperature but leftovers may be refrigerated.

For the Vinaigrette Dressing;

▶ Blend ¼ cup vinegar (apple cider or red wine) with 2 tablespoons Dijon mustard, salt and pepper to taste. Add ¾ cups extra virgin olive oil and mix very well so that ingredients blend completely. Use a blender or mixer if desired. Add herbs and garlic as desired.

Servings: 6

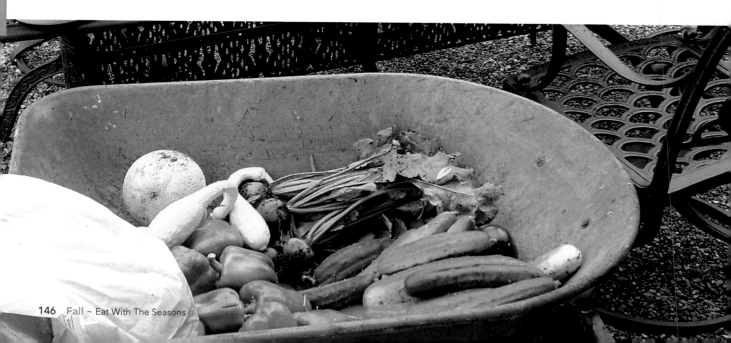

Harvest Squash Soup

This is a very hardy version of squash soup that serves as a meal along with some whole grain crusty bread and a nice green salad. The cilantro-lime sauce adds a nice zip!

- 2½ to 3 pounds butternut squash, peeled, seeds scooped out, and chopped
- 2 tablespoon organic butter, (or olive oil)
- 4 cloves garlic, peeled and smashed
- 1 medium onion, chopped
- 5 tablespoons quinoa, rinsed (you may substitute brown basmati rice if preferred)
- 2 medium carrots, sliced
- 2 tablespoons parsley, chopped
- 1 bay leaf
- 1 teaspoon cumin
- ½ teaspoon ground coriander
- Salt and freshly ground black pepper, to taste
- 8 cups water or stock

Cilantro Lime Sauce
- 1 cup greek yogurt
- 1 small jalapeño chile pepper, seeded and minced
- 2 tablespoons cilantro, chopped
- 2 limes, zest and juice
- ¼ teaspoon sea salt

▶ In a soup pot, melt the butter (or olive oil), over medium heat. Add the onion, squash, carrot, garlic, bay leaf, parsley, and quinoa; cook to soften the onion, stirring frequently, about 5 minutes. Add the spices, ½ teaspoon of salt, and some pepper and cook 5 minutes longer. Add the water, or stock, and bring to a boil, then lower the heat and simmer, partially covered, for about 25 minutes.

▶ While soup is cooking, make the Cilantro Lime Sauce by mixing all the ingredients together.

▶ Puree the soup with immersion blender or blender until smooth but leaving a little texture and flecks of squash, (or pass it through a food mill if you want a more refined soup). Taste for salt.

▶ Ladle it into bowls and serve with a spoonful of yogurt sauce on top.

Servings: 8

Leafy Greens Shepherd's Pie

The color orange reminds me of fall and I love to eat sweet potatoes in the fall. This mixture of leafy greens and sweet potatoes is perfect because the leafy greens give me the phytonutrients I need for energy and good blood, along with the vitamin A, potassium, protein, fiber, and loads of other nutrients in the sweet potato. How perfect!

- 2 pounds sweet potatoes, peeled and cut into 2-inch chunks
- 3 cloves of garlic
- 1 tablespoon sea salt
- Extra virgin olive oil
- 2 large onions, chopped
- 3 cloves garlic, minced
- ½ bunch collards, washed and chopped
- 1 bunch of kale, chopped
- 1 bunch Swiss chard or spinach, chopped
- 8 ounces vegetable broth
- Salt and pepper to taste

▶ In a large pot add about 6 cups water and the salt. Bring to a boil, add sweet potatoes and reduce heat and simmer until potatoes are tender. (Sweet potatoes can also be baked in a 350°F degree oven until soft.)

▶ Meanwhile in a large saucepan heat olive oil. Add onions, and cook for 3 minutes. Add collards and about 1 cup of the broth. Stir, cover and cook for about 10 minutes stirring occasionally. Add kale and more vegetable broth if necessary. Cover again and steam for about 8 minutes, or until kale is almost cooked. Stir. Add Swiss chard or spinach, garlic, pepper and salt and stir until wilted and most of the liquid is evaporated. Remove from heat. Taste for seasonings and adjust.

▶ Using a slotted spoon, transfer the vegetables to an olive oil coated casserole dish.
Top with Gruyère cheese (or feta if you prefer).

▶ Drain the potatoes when finished, reserving ⅓ cup of the liquid, and return to pot. Mash the potatoes until smooth using the liquid, and add salt, pepper, garlic powder if desired and olive oil to taste. Spread the mashed potatoes over the vegetables. Sprinkle with a pinch of nutmeg and a good olive oil. Set the broiler on high. Broil until lightly browned and heated through.

Servings: 8

MILLET & SWEET POTATO BURGERS

This is a nice change from the bean burgers that I often make and can be made with leftover millet and sweet potatoes for a quick dinner. Although there are lots of ingredients, it's all made in the food processor.

- 1 cup dried millet
- 1 large sweet potato, or yam, peeled and chopped
- 1 medium onion, chopped
- 3 cups water
- 1 cup chickpeas, cooked
- ⅛ cup tamari or shoyu
- 1 teaspoon olive oil
- 1 medium carrot, grated

- ½ cup sunflower seeds
- 1 teaspoon cumin
- 1 teaspoon coriander
- 1 teaspoon fennel seeds
- ½ teaspoon freshly ground pepper
- ¼ teaspoon cayenne pepper
- 1 tablespoon brown rice flour
- ¼ cup fresh parsley, chopped

▶ Preheat the oven to 400°F.

▶ Rinse the millet in a fine sieve. Place in a deep skillet over medium heat with the chopped sweet potato (or yam), onions, and water (or veggie broth). Simmer covered for about 30 minutes, or until both the millet and the sweet potato are soft and the liquid has cooked out.

▶ Place in a food processor and add the chickpeas, carrot and sunflower seeds; pulse together until chunky. Add the tamari, olive oil, cumin, coriander, fennel, pepper, cayenne, brown rice flour, and parsley; blend well. Add salt and pepper to taste.

▶ For 6 patties, scoop about 8 ounces each and place on a baking sheet lined with parchment paper. Spray lightly with olive oil. Bake in the oven for 20 minutes, until golden brown.

Servings: 6

PEPPERY PARSNIP FRIES

Here is another way to eat yummy parsnips which are loaded with silicon which is necessary for rebuilding connective tissue and essential for proper calcium absorption. Because of the silicon, these white, carrot looking vegetables are great for building bone strength, calming an aggravated liver, and improving digestion. So easy to make!

- 8 medium parsnips, peeled
- 1 tablespoon olive oil
- ¼ cup grated Parmesan cheese
- ½ teaspoon salt and freshly ground black pepper
- ⅛ teaspoon ground nutmeg

▶ Cut parsnips lengthwise into 2½-inch x ½-inch sticks. In a large re-sealable plastic bag, combine the oil, Parmesan cheese, salt, pepper and nutmeg. Add parsnips, a few sticks at a time, and shake to coat.

▶ Line two 15x10x1-inch baking pans with foil; coat the foil with non-stick cooking spray. Place parsnips in a single layer in pans. Bake at 425º F for 20 to 25 minutes or until tender, turning several times.

Servings: 8

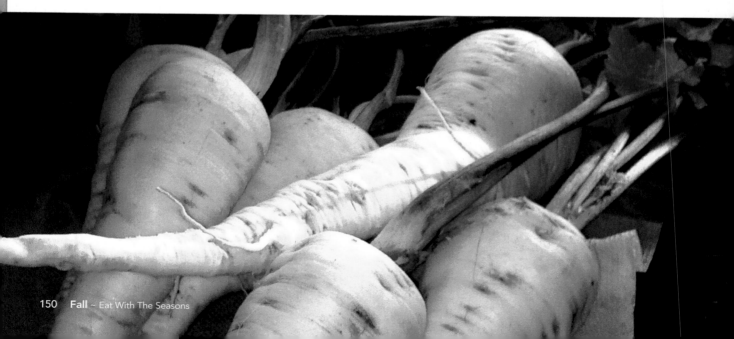

POLENTA PIZZA

*Although homemade polenta can be a bit time consuming to make, it is one of my favorite things to eat.
I always feel like I'm at a 4 star restaurant when I treat myself to this easy recipe. Once made there are so many
possibilities for it. Try this pizza with the roasted vegetables, and use any vegetables you have in your refrigerator.*

- 2 teaspoons extra virgin olive oil
- 1 onion chopped
- 1 teaspoon oregano (1 tablespoon fresh)
- 1 teaspoon basil (1 tablespoon fresh)
- 1 small zucchini, diced
- ½ eggplant, diced
- 1½ cups tomato sauce
- 3 cups water, boiling
- 1 teaspoon salt
- 1 teaspoon olive oil
- 1 cup polenta
- 1 teaspoon sea salt, or to taste
- ¼ cup Parmesan cheese
- 8 tablespoons grated mozzarella cheese or goat cheese or feta (optional) for topping

▶ Preheat oven to 350°F.

▶ Heat 2 teaspoons olive oil in skillet. Sauté onion until soft. Add garlic and herbs; sauté a few minutes more.

▶ Dice zucchini and eggplant.

▶ Put vegetable mixture and tomato sauce in a pot and simmer for one hour.

▶ Prepare the polenta. Bring water to a boil, add salt and oil. Slowly add polenta, stirring continuously with a whisk. Lower heat and continue stirring for 10 to15 minutes until mixture can hold the spoon upright on its own. Mix in Parmesan cheese and salt to taste.

▶ Lightly oil a 10-inch pie plate or 8x8-inch pan. Pour polenta into pan and smooth the top. Bake for 30 minutes.

▶ Spoon tomato mixture on top of the baked polenta. Cut into slices and serve with grated cheese on top if desired.

Servings: 8

Quinoa Minestrone Soup

I found this recipe when I was in California working with an associate of mine. We made it one evening to test it on her children and it was a big hit. Since then it has become a big part of my soup repertoire.

- 2 tablespoons olive oil
- 2 medium carrots, diced
- 1 cup fennel, cut into ½-inch dice
- 1 cup red onion, diced
- 2 large cloves garlic, minced
- 2 bay leaves
- 2 teaspoons fresh thyme leaves or ½ teaspoon dried
- ¼ teaspoon fennel seeds, crushed

- 1½ cups cooked cannellini beans, drained (and rinsed if using canned)
- 2 cups plum tomatoes, diced
- ⅓ cup uncooked quinoa, rinsed and drained
- Sea salt and fresh ground pepper to taste
- 1 cup fresh baby spinach
- 3 tablespoons fresh basil leaves, thinly sliced
- 2 ounces Parmigiano-Reggiano cheese, grated (about ½ cup), optional

▶ In a large heavy-bottomed pot or Dutch oven, heat oil over medium heat. Add carrots, fennel, onion, garlic, bay leaves, thyme, and fennel seeds. Cook, stirring often, until vegetables are tender, about 8 minutes.

▶ Add 6 cups water, beans, tomatoes and quinoa. Increase heat to high and bring to a boil. Reduce heat to low and simmer gently until quinoa is tender, about 20 minutes.

▶ Remove bay leaves and season with salt and pepper. Stir spinach and basil into soup about 4 minutes before serving.

▶ Garnish each bowl with cheese.

Servings: 8

Roasted Cauliflower

This cool weather vegetable is another member of the cruciferous vegetable group with all the cancer fighting, liver enhancing, detoxifying properties of kale and cabbage. Most of the recipes I find for cauliflower contain lots of cheese and cream, but not this one. I find this so delicious that it doesn't last long enough to save for leftovers.

- 1 head cauliflower, cored and cut into florets
- 2 tablespoons olive oil
- 3 tablespoons tamari soy sauce
- 1 clove garlic, minced (or use garlic powder)

- 1 teaspoon red pepper flakes
- Salt and pepper to taste
- Optional cilantro for garnish

▶ In a bowl or a ziploc bag, place all the ingredients except salt and pepper. Blend together well and place on a baking sheet covered with parchment paper. Bake in 350°F oven for 25 minutes or until tender.

▶ Remove from oven. Add pepper and salt if needed. Top with chopped cilantro if desired and serve.

Servings: 6

ROASTED SQUASH SOUP

The depth of flavor in this soup comes from the roasting of the squashes and onions which brings out the sweetness of the flavors. The fact that squashes and pumpkins are high in Vitamin A and C, Potassium, Manganese and Omega 3's is just an added bonus. These high antioxidant, anti-cancer foods are known to help regulate blood sugar balance as well. What more does anyone need to make these ingredients a favorite fall and winter staple?

- 1 large butternut squash, cut in half and seeded (save the seeds)
- 6 cloves garlic, unpeeled
- 3 large red onions, peeled and cut into quarters
- 1 teaspoon sea salt
- Freshly ground pepper
- 12 cloves garlic, peeled and left whole

- 2 tablespoons fresh rosemary, chopped and divided
- 2 tablespoons fresh thyme leaves, divided
- 4½ to 6 cups vegetable stock or chicken stock
- 2 tablespoons balsamic vinegar
- 1 tablespoon black strap molasses
- ½ cup plain yogurt or grated Gruyère cheese

▶ Preheat the oven to 400°F and adjust the racks to allow squash to sit on the lower rack and the onions on the top rack.

▶ Cut squash in half, scoop out the seeds and put aside. Prick the squash, rub the inside with olive oil and place squash-side down on a shallow baking dish/pan. Stuff 3 garlic cloves under each cavity. Bake on the lower oven rack for about 45 minutes. Test by inserting a sharp knife into the flesh. Let cool enough to handle.

▶ Meanwhile, in a large bowl, toss the onions with oil, salt and pepper. Spread on a lightly oiled baking sheet (or on parchment paper), and bake on the top rack in the preheated oven for 20 minutes. Remove from oven and stir the onions. Add the garlic and sprinkle 1 tablespoon each of rosemary and thyme over the top. Return to the oven and roast for another 20 minutes or until vegetables are very soft and golden brown. Set aside.

▶ When squash is cool enough to handle, scoop out the flesh. In a food processor, blend roughly 1 cup of the squash, 1 cup onion mixture, ½ cup stock, vinegar, molasses and remaining rosemary and thyme. Transfer the mixture to a large saucepan. Repeat with the remaining 2 batches of 1 cup onion, 1 cup squash, ½ cup stock. (If your food processor is large enough you may adjust this to fewer steps.) *Note: the puree may be frozen at this point or refrigerated until ready to serve for up to 2 days.*

▶ When ready to serve, in a large saucepan bring purée to a gentle simmer over medium heat. Stir in 3- to 4½ cups of the remaining stock, 1 cup at a time, until the desired consistency is achieved. Blend well and heat through. Test for seasonings. Serve warm and garnish with shredded Gruyère cheese or a dollop of plain yogurt.

Servings: 6

ROASTED SQUASH WITH GARLIC & PARSLEY

Here's an easier version of roasted squash that combines some of my favorite flavors together. You can use any of the winter squashes that you like. The easiest to peel is the butternut.

- 1 large, or 2 small winter squashes, peeled, seeded and cut into 1-inch pieces
- 2 tablespoons extra virgin olive oil, divided
- 1½ teaspoon sea salt
- 3 cloves garlic, minced
- 2 tablespoons fresh parsley, chopped

▶ Preheat the oven to 375°F. Cover baking sheet with parchment paper.

▶ Toss the squash with 1 tablespoon of olive oil, salt, and ¼ teaspoon pepper. Spread on baking sheet, roast, stirring occasionally, until tender throughout and lightly browned, about 30 minutes depending on the type of squash.

▶ Heat the remaining olive oil in a small skillet over medium heat. Add the garlic and cook, stirring, until fragrant, about 30 seconds to a minute. Be careful not to brown as the garlic will taste bitter. Toss the squash with the garlic and parsley, adjust seasonings and serve.

Servings: 8

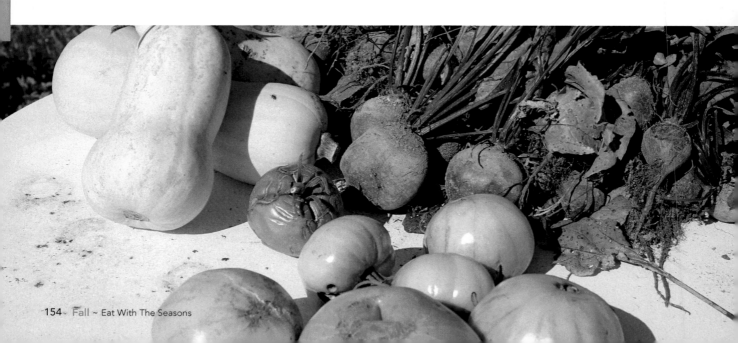

Turkey Quinoa Meatloaf

This is a healthy staple that I love because it gives me so much mileage. I usually save quinoa from another meal to turn this into a quick dinner.

- ¼ cup quinoa
- ½ cup water
- 1 teaspoon olive oil
- 1 small onion, chopped
- 1 large clove garlic, chopped
- 20 ounces ground turkey
- 1 tablespoon tomato paste
- 1 tablespoon hot pepper sauce
- 2 tablespoons tamari sauce
- 1 medium egg beaten
- ½ teaspoon sea salt
- 1 teaspoon freshly ground black pepper

Topping
- 2 tablespoons Dijon mustard
- 2 teaspoons tamari sauce
- 2 teaspoons tomato paste
- 1 teaspoon water

▶ Bring the quinoa and water to a boil in a saucepan over high heat. Reduce heat to medium-low, cover, and simmer until the quinoa is tender and the water has been absorbed, about 15 to 20 minutes. Set aside.

▶ Preheat an oven to 350°F.

▶ Heat the olive oil in a skillet over medium heat. Stir in the onion; cook and stir until the onion has softened and turned translucent, about 5 minutes. Add the garlic and cook for another minute; remove from heat to cool.

▶ Stir the turkey, cooked quinoa, onions, tomato paste, hot sauce, 2 tablespoons tamari, egg, salt, and pepper in a large bowl until well combined. The mixture will be very moist. Shape into a loaf on a foil lined baking sheet. Combine the Dijon mustard, 2 teaspoons tamari, 2 teaspoons tomato paste, and 1 teaspoon water in a small bowl. Rub the paste over the top of the meatloaf.

▶ Bake in the preheated oven until no longer pink in the center, about 50 minutes. An instant-read thermometer inserted into the center should read at least 160°F. Let the meatloaf cool for 10 minutes before slicing and serving.

Servings: 8

Vegetable & Bulgur Chili

This recipe is a staple for our Thanksgiving bonfire night because we have so many vegetarians in our family. No one ever seems to know the difference because of the bold flavor and texture of the bulgur wheat. Once we add our favorite toppings it's even more delicious!

- ¾ cup whole grain bulgur wheat
- 1 cup boiling water
- 1 cup vegetable broth, heated to almost boiling
- 1½ cups green and red pepper, finely chopped
- 1 large onion, chopped
- 2 cups zucchini, chopped
- 1 cup celery, chopped
- 2 medium carrots, chopped
- 2 tablespoons olive oil
- 1 can (14-ounce) diced tomatoes
- 2 cups tomato juice, all natural, low sodium
- 1 can tomato sauce
- 1 can (16-ounce) pinto beans, drained and rinsed
- 1 can (16-ounce) kidney beans, drained and rinsed
- 1 cup veggie broth
- 3 tablespoon chili powder, or to taste
- 2 large garlic cloves, minced
- ½ teaspoon ground cumin
- ¼ teaspoon cayenne pepper, or to taste

▶ Rinse the bulgur and place it in a bowl; stir in the boiling water and the heated veggie broth. Cover and let stand for 30 minutes or until most of the liquid is absorbed. Drain and squeeze dry.

▶ In a large Dutch oven, sauté the green and red peppers, onions, zucchini, carrots, and celery in olive oil until tender, about 6 minutes. Stir in the canned tomatoes and mix. Cook a few minutes more. Add in bulgur, tomato juice, tomato sauce, beans, veggie broth, chili powder, garlic, cumin and cayenne. Bring to a boil. Reduce heat; cover and simmer for about 20 to 25 minutes or until heated through.

▶ Use your favorite chili toppings for serving, such as, shredded cheese, yogurt, scallions or onions, salsa, etc.

Servings: 8

WHEAT BERRY-CRANBERRY SALAD

I learned this recipe from a friend who has helped me with many a cooking class. It's always a hit when I bring it to fall gatherings. It tastes great as a salad but may also be used as a stuffing for fall squashes like acorn or butternut. The cranberries add just enough tartness to balance the sweet. People are not always familiar with the whole grain form of wheat (wheat berries), and it has a nice poppy flavor. You can find it with the other grains in the grocery store. A little bit goes a long way and it's important to really chew each mouthful for good digestion.

- 1½ cups uncooked wheat berries
- 1 teaspoon salt
- 1 strip of kombu* (seaweed)
- 2 cups fresh cranberries
- ¼ cup maple syrup
- ¼ cup cranberry juice
- 4 tablespoons olive oil
- 2 tablespoons raspberry or white wine vinegar
- 3 teaspoons Dijon mustard
- ¼ teaspoon freshly ground black pepper
- ½ cup diced celery
- ½ cup thinly sliced green onions
- ⅓ cup chopped fresh parsley
- ⅓ cup chopped pecans, toasted
- Feta or goat cheese for topping

▶ Place the wheat berries in a medium bowl and cover with water to 2-inches above the wheat berries. Cover and let stand overnight. Drain

▶ Place wheat berries and ½ teaspoon salt in a medium saucepan. Cover with water and bring to a boil. Cover, add 1 strip kombu, reduce heat and cook 1 hour or until tender (the wheat berries will be tender and have a little pop to them). Drain, remove kombu and cool to room temperature.

▶ Combine cranberries and maple syrup in a small saucepan over medium heat; bring to a boil. Cook for about 4 minutes or until cranberries pop, stirring often (If using dried cranberries then cook until they are soft and plump, and have absorbed the maple syrup). Transfer to a large bowl; cool 10 minutes.

▶ Add juice, vinegar, olive oil, mustard, pepper, and remaining ½ teaspoon salt to cranberry mixture; stir well to combine. Add wheat berries, celery, onion, parsley and pecans to cranberry mixture; stir well. Serve at room temperature or cover and chill.

▶ Top with crumbled feta or goat cheese if desired.

Servings: 10
Kombu can be found in health food stores or ordered online. See Resources page 248.

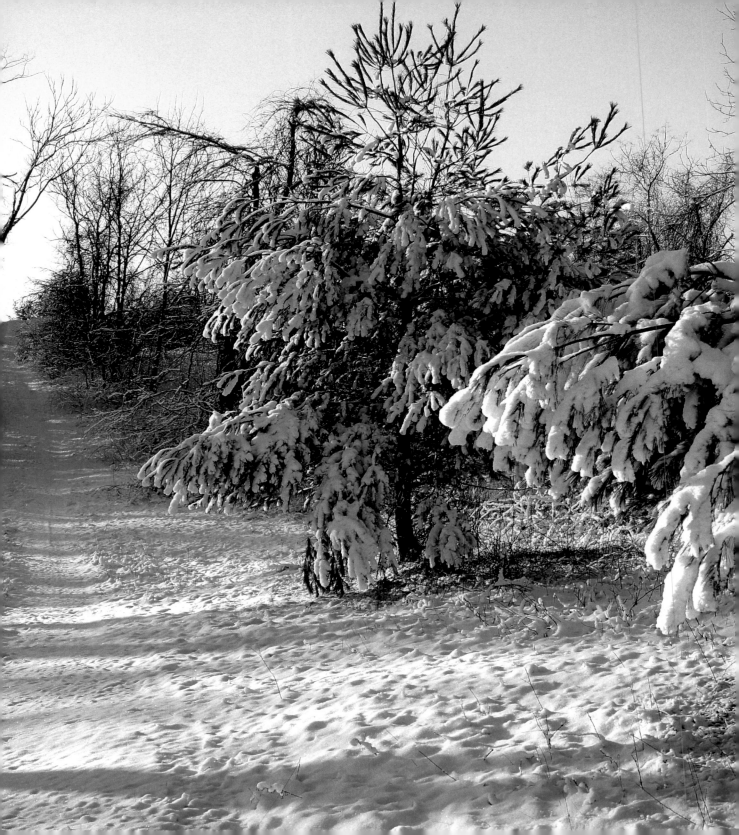

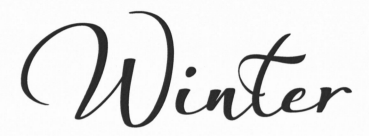

An old Ayurvedic saying is,
"You are what you digest."

Shifting Into Winter

The stillness of winter has a language all its own. The voice of nature is a silent purity that expresses the moving inward, the dying of the old, the hibernation of plants and animals that brings out the voice of silence. The quiet stillness permeates the air as though a veil has settled over the earth to hush the noise. When I go walking at this time of year, I love that hushed stillness as it soothes my soul. With the leaves off the trees, I can peer into the woods to see the streams and the animals and there is more depth and expanse to the view.

The Holidays bring a change from orange and browns to red and green and blue. Twinkle lights appear to help us feel warm and fuzzy and bring light to all the long dark days. There's a time of quiet celebration before we settle into the winter routine of inner growth. Winter Solstice occurs on December 21 and marks the longest night of the year. The sun reaches its most southern point in the sky at local noon. After this night the days start getting longer. It's a nice day to celebrate quietly and reflect on what the year has delivered and where one is in their acceptance and gratitude. With winter comes the longer nights and the colder days where we usually end up inside quite a bit. It is a time to be quiet, stay warm and rest more fully. This is the season when I take more time to develop my inner growth by reading meaningful books, meditating, writing, and thinking. It's the perfect time to bring out that inner creativity and watch it work. Doing outside activities in the cold weather helps me to stay healthy, builds my immune system, keeps my spine and joints flexible, and helps me feel refreshed. I find it very soothing to walk or snowshoe in the quiet winter woods.

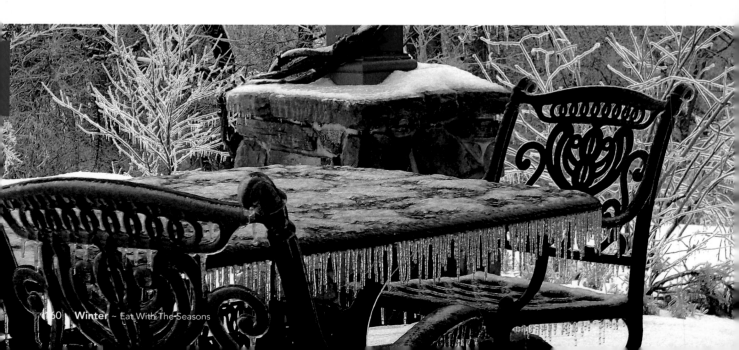

My thoughts on shifting...INNER WARMTH, REST, SPIRITUAL GROWTH

Winter is the end of all the seasons. Our diet needs to shift to reflect this weather and it's a good time to eat heavier foods and more good fats. We love to hear about warm, hearty soups and stews, roasted root vegetables, and hot oatmeal with cinnamon. Foods need to be cooked longer and slower, with less water and at lower temperatures. Slow cookers work so well in this season as does roasting! This is also the time to eat more bitter foods like; turnips, celery, escarole, endive, oats, quinoa, and watercress. Citrus peel is also bitter, as well as herbs like chicory root, burdock root and horsetail. Try adding these to your tea. It is also the season of salty taste to bring body heat deeper into the body. Cook with seaweeds, miso, soy, sea salt, barley and millet. As Paul Pitchford says, "Use small regular amounts in winter to nurture deep inner experiences and preserve joy in the heart." According to Chinese physiology the element of winter is water. This is the "essential medium of the body through which all things pass...People with deficient water energy may find it difficult to slow down, relax, or rest, and an inability to reflect clearly." (Elson Haas) The organ associated with the season is the kidney which in turn affects the bladder, ears, and adrenal glands. The kidneys are the root of the body, providing energy and warmth. They filter the blood and keep the body clean and in balance and as such govern our life force. It is the seat of willpower, generates ambition and the desire to do something with one's life. (Haas). Kidney imbalances can show up in bone problems (especially knees, lower back, teeth), hearing loss and ear infections, head/hair problems like hair loss and premature graying, urinary, sexual, and reproductive imbalances, poor growth and development of mind and body, and, excessive fear and insecurity. (Paul Pitchford) The water element emotion is fear and "fear is deeply rooted". In Chinese medicine it is said that excessive fear and general insecurity about life can injure the kidneys, or, weak kidneys generate fearful feelings and block loving experiences. "By restoring the kidneys to any significant degree, one typically feels a tremendous elation as the dark cloud of fear lifts."(Pitchford)

Winter Seasonal Plan

BREAKFAST OPTIONS: What winter options would you like to add to your breakfast routine? Try the heartier warm cereals like oats or buckwheat with almond milk and dried fruit, nuts and cinnamon to keep you warm and satisfied. Eat lots of citrus to keep up the vitamin C. Write down your fall breakfast choices here:

_____

SNACK OPTIONS: Keep good breakfast bars with dried fruit, nuts and seeds in your snack choices, along with cooked fruit like applesauce or sweet cooked root vegetables. Nuts and seeds are a good choice for the healthy fats that give warmth and energy in cold weather. What are your winter snack choices? Write them here:

_____

LUNCH: What are your all time favorites? List these here. Now add in some choices that are seasonal. As the days are shorter and colder make lots of warming soups and stews to keep you satisfied. Eat your heavier proteins and fats in this season with lots of garlic and onions to fight virus. Add broccoli, walnuts, and apples to your salads, along with fresh sauerkraut and coleslaws. Remember to cook extra at dinner to bring for next day lunches. Write your lunchtime choices here:

_____

MENTAL RECIPE FILE: Go through your mental recipe file and think back to meals you like to make in the winter. Which old stand by's would you like to keep that are still working for you? Write those here:

_____

NEW WINTER OPTIONS: Now, take a look at the menus in this chapter. Which recipes sound good to you? Choose 3-5 recipes and work with them this winter. Make them your own by working with the ingredients to create a meal that is satisfying to your needs. Write the recipe names here:

_____

WINTER EXERCISE: What changes are you going to make to your winter routine to help you flow with the season? The colder weather does not mean you have to stay inside. Why not try a winter activity like hiking or snowshoeing, if there's snow. It will help to keep you warmer and all you need is warm clothing. Continue to take walks outside on nice days to replenish Vitamin D that you lose when you don't get sunshine. Have you been intending to try a new activity? Why not put it in your schedule and try it out? Write your exercise commitments here:

_____

_____

_____

YOUR WINTER CIRCLE OF LIFE

Your life at this moment is a direct result of your actions over the last months and years.

This exercise will help you to discover which nourishment you are missing most. The Circle of Life has ten sections. Look at each section of the circle and place a dot on the line to designate how satisfied you are at this moment with this area of your life. A dot placed at the center of the circle, close to the middle, indicates dissatisfaction, while a dot placed on the periphery indicates ultimate happiness. Once you have placed a dot in each category, you connect the dots to see your current circle of life. Now you have a clear visual of any imbalances of nourishment, and a starting point for determining where you may wish to spend more time and energy to create balance. Pick the top three areas, circle them and write them down at the bottom of the page. Ask yourself, what's one thing I can do this season to move me in a more joyful direction for this category? Write it down for each category and get started by meditating on the action each day. Ask yourself, What am I putting off? Why? How am I giving back?

*See the chapter, HOW TO BEGIN, for more explanation of each category

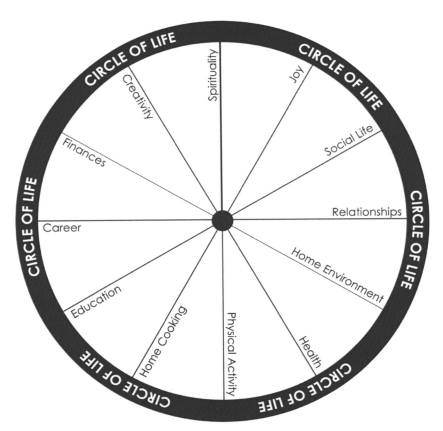

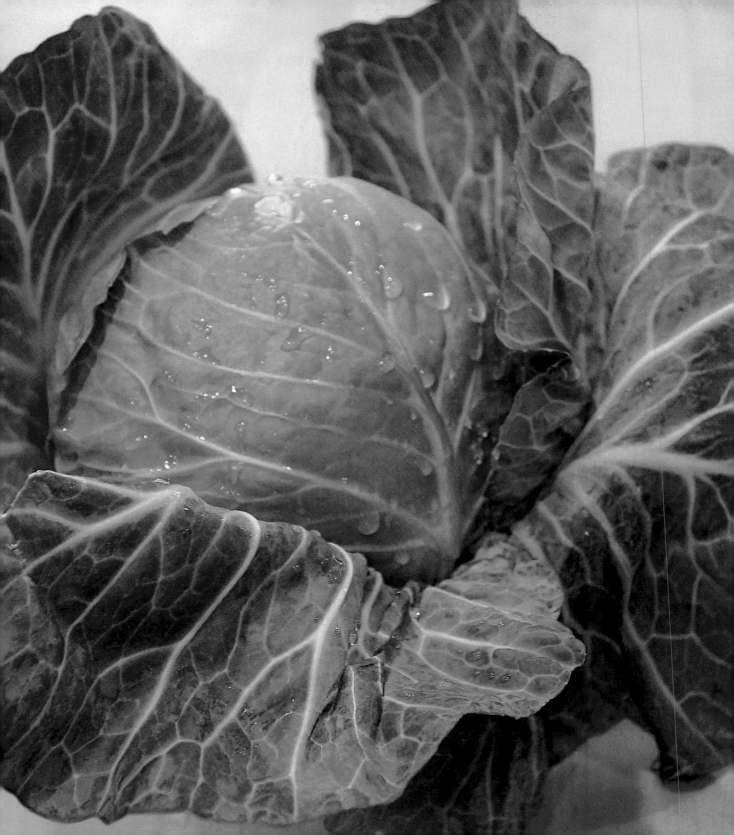

Winter Menus

MENU 1: Carrot Salad, Quinoa Minestrone Soup, Whole Grain Bread, Escarole Salad

MENU 2: Fresh Sauerkraut, Chermoula Baked Tempeh, Greens Sautéed in Olive Oil

MENU 3: Winter Mushroom Stew over Polenta or Mashed Potatoes, String Beans

MENU 4: Baked Beans with Miso & Apple Butter, Cilantro Lime Rice, Broccoli Apple Salad

MENU 5: Moroccan Style Tagine with Whole Wheat Couscous, Warm Sesame Greens

MENU 6: Celery Root Salad, Balsamic glazed Beets, Greek Bison Burgers

MENU 7: Millet & Sweet Potato Patties with Herbed Yogurt-Tofu, Crusty Beans and Kale

MENU 8: Barley Porcini Soup, Cornbread, Escarole Salad

MENU 9: Roasted Root Vegetables, Broiled Salmon, Kale with Feta and Olives

MENU 10: Turkey Quinoa Meatloaf, Brussels Sprouts & Cauliflower, Sweet Carrots

MENU 11: Vegetable Bulgur Chili with toppings of Greek Yogurt & Scallions, Cornbread, Green Salad

MENU 12: Wheat Berry Cranberry Salad, Peppery Parsnip Fries, Garlic Gingered Broccoli

A nice escarole salad is a great way to end any of these meals in the winter months. Escarole has a nice bitter crunchy flavor that can help stimulate the kidneys. Top off your meal with a fresh orange and you'll get your daily dose of Vitamin C. How perfect!

Baked Beans With
Miso & Apple Butter

This recipe is from my mentor Annemarie Colbin. It's very hearty for a warming fall or winter dish. Miso is a wonderful food to add to the diet. The basic ingredient is fermented soy paste combined with a grain, and it serves as a wonderful probiotic with lots of active enzymes. It can aid in digestion and is known to have anti-microbial properties.

- 2 cups dried kidney beans, soaked
- 6 cups water
- 1 strip kombu
- 1½ tablespoon mellow barley miso
- ¼ cup unsweetened and un-spiced apple butter
- 1½ teaspoon whole grain mustard
- 1 tablespoon grated onion
- ⅔ tablespoon brown rice vinegar

▶ Drain the beans and place in a 4-quart pot. Add the 6 cups of water and kombu and cook, covered, over low heat until tender, about 40 to 45 minutes. Remove kombu, drain, reserving 1 cup of the cooking liquid.

▶ Preheat the oven to 350°F. Oil a heavy 3-quart casserole or bean pot.

▶ In a medium bowl, combine the reserved bean-cooking liquid and the miso, apple butter, mustard, onion, and brown rice vinegar.

▶ Place the cooked beans in the pot, add the miso-apple butter mixture and stir to combine. Cover and bake for 1½ hours checking to make sure there is enough liquid and the beans do not dry out. Serve hot.

Servings: 8

BARLEY PORCINI SOUP

I love the combination of barley and mushrooms. I think that the Porcini mushroom water really gives this such a nice complex flavor that I don't need to add any beef to give the broth depth.

- ½ cup pearl barley, rinsed
- 4½ cups mushroom broth or chicken broth
- 1 ounce dried Porcini mushroom
- 2 cups boiling water
- 1 teaspoon butter
- 2 tablespoons olive oil
- 1 cup shallots, about 4, minced
- 8 cups white mushrooms (about 20 ounces), sliced
- 2 stalks celery, finely chopped

- 1 tablespoon fresh sage (or 1 teaspoon dried Herbes de Provençe), minced
- ½ teaspoon sea salt
- ½ teaspoon freshly ground pepper
- 2 tablespoons tomato paste
- 1 cup red wine
- ½ cup Greek yogurt (optional)
- ¼ cup chives, minced

▶ Combine barley and 1½ cups broth in a small saucepan. Bring to a boil over high heat; cover, reduce heat to low and simmer until the barley is tender, 30 to 35 minutes.

▶ Meanwhile, combine porcini mushrooms and boiling water in a medium bowl and let soak until the mushrooms are soft, about 20 minutes. Line a sieve with paper towels, set over a bowl and pour mushrooms and soaking liquid through it. Reserve the soaking liquid. Transfer the mushrooms to a cutting board and finely chop.

▶ Heat butter and oil in a Dutch oven over medium-high heat. Add shallots and cook, stirring often, until softened, about 2 minutes. Add white mushrooms and cook, stirring often, until they have released their juices and started to brown, 8 to 10 minutes. Add the porcini mushrooms, celery, sage or herbs, salt, and pepper and cook, stirring often, until beginning to soften, about 3 minutes. Add tomato paste and mix well.

▶ Add wine and cook, scraping up any browned bits with a wooden spoon, until most the wine has evaporated, about 1 minute.

▶ Add the soaking liquid and the remaining 3 cups of broth, increase heat to high and bring to a boil. Reduce heat and simmer, stirring occasionally, until the celery is tender and the soup has thickened, about 18 to 22 minutes.

▶ Add the cooked barley and continue cooking, stirring occasionally, until heated through, about 5 minutes. Top with yogurt if desired. Garnish with chives.

Servings: 4

BROCCOLI & APPLE SALAD

I like this salad as a side dish for fall or winter because it adds a fresh flavor to many of the cooked stews and soups that make up my winter diet. It tastes good topped with chopped walnuts. Broccoli is high in antioxidants and sulfur compounds, which are known to help fight cancer.

- 6 tablespoons apple cider vinegar
- 2 tablespoons Dijon-style mustard
- 1 tablespoon Extra virgin olive oil
- 1 tablespoon honey, if desired
- ½ teaspoon freshly ground black pepper
- ¼ teaspoon sea salt
- 1¼ cups Granny Smith apple, chopped
- ¼ cup walla walla or Vidalia onion, minced
- 1 head broccoli, blanched for 1 minute and coarsely chopped

▶ Combine the first 6 ingredients in a large bowl and mix well with a whisk.

▶ Place the chopped broccoli in a bowl with the vinegar mixture. Add the chopped apples and minced onion, tossing to coat.

▶ Serve at room temperature.

Servings: 8 / Yield: 4 cup

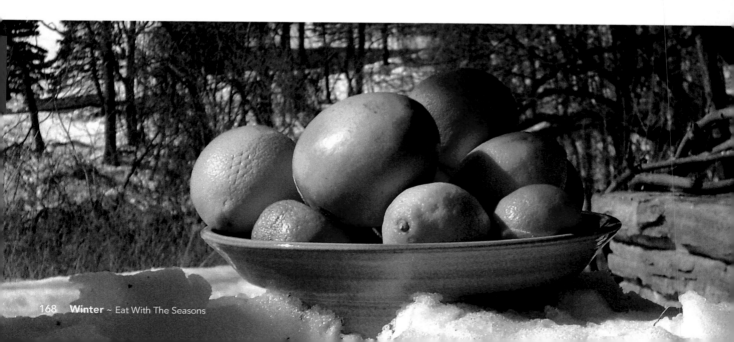

CHARMOULA BAKED TEMPEH

Charmoula is a great Moroccan marinade for things like fish, tempeh, or lamb. It's a wonderfully spicy Moroccan flavoring. I learned this recipe from Chef Peter Berley when I studied at The Natural Gourmet Institute and was very surprised at how much I loved it.

- ½ cup extra virgin olive oil
- ½ cup fresh cilantro, chopped
- ⅓ cup lemon juice, freshly squeezed
- 2 cloves garlic, roughly chopped
- 2½ teaspoons coarse sea salt or kosher salt
- 2 teaspoons paprika
- 2 teaspoons cumin seeds
- 1 teaspoon coriander seed
- ½ teaspoon cayenne pepper
- 2 pkgs (8-ounce each) soy tempeh, cut into 1-inch cubes

▶ To prepare the charmoula for the tempeh, in a medium bowl, whisk 1¼ cups of water with the oil, cilantro, lemon juice, garlic, and salt. In a spice blender, grind the paprika, cumin, coriander, and cayenne. Whisk the ground spices into the olive oil mixture.

▶ In a large skillet or sauté pan, arrange the tempeh squares in one layer. Pour the spice mixture over the tempeh. Pour the spice mixture over the tempeh. Over high heat, bring the mixture to a simmer. Reduce the heat, cover, and simmer until most, but not all, of the liquid is absorbed, about 15 minutes. If it looks too dry, add a little more water.

Servings: 8

Creamy Swiss Chard & Potato Soup

Inspired by Chef Peter Berley, this is another version of the Potato Leek Soup except that this one has caraway seeds in it. These, along with spices like cumin, help us to better digest sulfurous vegetables like the turnips and cabbage.

- 2 tablespoons unsalted butter
- 1 tablespoon olive oil
- 2 medium leeks, white and light green parts only, rinsed and coarsely chopped
- 1 teaspoon sea salt
- 4 cloves garlic, chopped
- 2 teaspoons caraway seeds
- 3 small white turnips, cut into ¾-inch pieces
- 4 to 5 potatoes, (Yukon gold, or large red), peeled and cut into 1-inch pieces
- 1 bunch Swiss Chard, trimmed and chopped
- Freshly ground black pepper

▶ In a large saucepan over medium heat, melt the butter and mix with olive oil. Add the leeks, season with a little salt, and sauté until soft but not browned, about 3 minutes. Add the garlic and caraway seeds and sauté for 1 more minute.

▶ Add 6 cups of water, or vegetable broth, the turnips, and potatoes, and bring to a boil over high heat. Add the 1 teaspoon of salt, reduce the heat to medium, and simmer, covered, until the vegetables are tender, about 10 to 15 minutes.

▶ Add the chard and simmer until wilted, 2 to 3 more minutes. Using an immersion blender, or in the blender in batches, blend the soup until creamy. Season with salt and lots of pepper and serve.
Try serving with a dollop of Greek yogurt.

Servings: 6

CRUSTY WHITE BEANS & KALE

This is so delicious that I have to stop myself from eating too much. I love it topped with umeboshi plum vinegar but many other vinegars taste great too. I love to make it in my cast iron skillet.

- 2 cans (15-ounce each) cannellini beans, rinsed and drained
- 3 tablespoons olive oil, or clarified butter, or a mix
- Fine-grain sea salt
- 1 medium onion chopped
- 4 cloves garlic, minced
- 1 bunch Kale, Swiss Chard, or spinach, leaves cut into ribbons
- Freshly ground black pepper and sea salt to taste
- Extra virgin olive oil, for drizzling
- Freshly grated Parmesan cheese
- Umeboshi plum vinegar, optional

▶ Heat olive oil and/or butter over medium heat in a very wide skillet. Add the beans to the hot pan in a single layer. If you don't have a big-enough skillet, just do the sauté step in two batches. Stir to coat the beans with olive oil, then let them sit long enough to brown on one side, about 3 or 4 minutes, before turning to brown on the other side, also about 3 or 4 minutes. The beans should be golden and a bit crunchy on the outside and soft and creamy on the inside.

▶ Salt to taste, then add the onion and garlic and cook for 1 to 2 minutes, until the onion softens.

▶ In a separate pan, steam the greens until wilted. Drain the water and add the chard, kale, or spinach to the bean mixture. Mix well. Remove from the heat and season to taste with a generous dose of salt and pepper. Drizzle with a bit of top-quality extra virgin olive oil, 1 tablespoon of umeboshi plum vinegar, and sprinkle with freshly grated Parmesan. Enjoy!

Servings: 10

GARLIC SOUP

This is such a nice warming soup for the winter months, or when you feel a cold coming on. Garlic is one of those whole foods that contain sulfur compounds (like cabbage and eggs) and promotes antioxidant activity. That means it helps to fight colds and sickness! It is also known for its powerful antiviral and antimicrobial properties, which serve to fight off viruses. This is a great choice to begin every meal in the winter, and so easy to make.

- 5 cups water
- 6 large garlic cloves, minced or put through a press
- 1 to 2 teaspoon sea salt, to taste
- ½ teaspoon dried thyme
- 4 fresh sage leaves, chopped, or ½ teaspoon dried
- 1 bay leaf
- 2 tablespoons fresh parsley, chopped

▶ Bring the water to a boil and add the garlic, salt, thyme, sage, and bay leaf. Simmer 15 minutes. Adjust seasonings.

▶ Serve at once, topping each with parsley.

Servings: 4

HIJIKI SALAD

This is a delicious little salad that I learned from another chef while giving a class together. Seaweed is a wonder food that is so under-used in our cooking.

- ⅔ cup hijiki soaked for 15 minutes and drained
- 1 teaspoon olive oil
- 2 tablespoons umeboshi vinegar
- 1 medium grated beet
- ½ cup walnuts
- Mixed greens

▶ Sauté hijiki in oil for 20 minutes (or cook in water).

▶ Allow to cool.

▶ Mix all ingredients together adding parsley and sea salt to taste.

▶ Serve on a bed of mixed lettuce

Servings: 4

MEDITERRANEAN LENTIL SOUP

Lentils have the added bonus of being much quicker to cook than beans, so no soaking is required. This nutritious soup has a bit of everything — leafy greens, starchy potatoes, antioxidant-rich tomatoes, not to mention those protein-rich lentils. Lentils are high in fiber and provide antioxidant protection and heart health.

- 1 tablespoon olive oil
- 1 medium yellow onion, cut into ¼-inch dice
- 1 celery rib, thinly sliced
- 2 small carrots, thinly sliced
- 2 cloves garlic, minced
- 1½ cup French green lentils, rinsed
- 3 cups blond chicken stock, mushroom or vegetable stock
- 1 bay leaf
- ½ teaspoon dried oregano
- ½ teaspoon dried basil

- ¼ teaspoon dried red pepper flakes
- 1 teaspoon salt
- ½ teaspoon freshly ground black pepper
- 1 can (14-ounce) diced tomatoes, with their juice
- 3 medium Yukon Gold potatoes, cubed
- 1 tablespoon fresh lemon juice, or 1 tablespoon red wine vinegar
- 2 cups (packed) fresh spinach or chard, well rinsed, stems removed and large leaves cut into 1-inch wide ribbons
- Freshly grated Parmesan cheese (optional), for garnish

▶ Heat the olive oil in a large, heavy pot over medium heat. Add the onion, celery and carrots and cook, stirring frequently for 5 minutes. Add the garlic and cook until the onion and garlic are soft but not browned, 1 minute longer.

▶ Add the lentils and stock. Increase the heat to high and bring to a boil. Reduce the heat to low and let simmer until the lentils soften, about 20 minutes.

▶ Add the bay leaf, oregano, basil, pepper flakes, salt, pepper, tomatoes, and potatoes. Let the soup simmer until the potatoes are tender, about 20 minutes longer.

▶ Just before serving, remove and discard the bay leaf. Add the lemon juice and spinach to the soup and let simmer gently, just until the spinach wilts, about 2 minutes (adding the lemon juice and greens just before serving helps the color of the greens stay bright). If you like a thinner soup, add more stock or some water. Serve the soup hot, garnished with Parmesan cheese, if desired.

Servings: 6

MOROCCAN-STYLE VEGETABLE TAGINE

A "tagine" is a Moroccan style slow-cooked stew braised at low temperatures. It's usually made in a special tajine pot. I really love the marinade for the tempeh and have used the same marinade for lamb and poultry. Although one of my more labor intensive recipes, it's so worth the effort. This is another adaptation of Chef Peter Berley. This is a wonderful dish to prepare ahead and let the flavors blend together before serving over a warm rice or whole wheat couscous.

Tempeh
- ½ cup extra virgin olive oil
- ½ cup water
- ⅓ cup parsley, finely chopped
- 6 tablespoons lemon juice, freshly squeezed
- 4 cloves garlic, crushed
- 2½ teaspoons sea salt
- 2 teaspoons ground cumin
- 2 teaspoons paprika
- ½ teaspoon cayenne pepper
- 1 pound tempeh, cut into 1-inch cubes

Tagine
- 2 tablespoons extra virgin olive oil
- 2 medium onions, diced
- 2 medium carrots, diced
- 2 stalks celery, diced
- 2 medium sweet potatoes, peeled and diced

- 2 cloves garlic, peeled and left whole
- 2 teaspoons sea salt
- 1 teaspoon cumin seeds
- 1 teaspoon caraway seeds
- 1 teaspoon coriander seed
- 1 small cinnamon stick
- ½ teaspoon paprika
- ½ teaspoon whole black peppercorn
- 3 cups cabbage, chopped
- 1½ cups water
- 1 cup tomatoes, peeled and chopped, with their juice

Garnish
- Chopped fresh cilantro
- Chopped fresh parsley
- Chives

▶ Adjust middle rack in oven and preheat to 350ºF.

▶ To prepare the tempeh: In a bowl, whisk together the oil, water, parsley, lemon juice, garlic, salt, cumin, paprika, and cayenne pepper.

▶ Arrange the tempeh cubes in a single layer in a baking dish. Pour on the marinade and cover securely with foil. Bake 35 to 40 minutes or until the tempeh has absorbed the marinade. Uncover and bake several minutes longer to brown.

▶ To prepare the tagine: In a 3-quart heavy bottomed Dutch oven over medium heat, warm the oil. Add the onions, carrots, celery, sweet potatoes, garlic, and salt. Turn the vegetables over in the oil with a wooden spoon, raise the heat, and bring to a simmer. Cover the pan, reduce heat to low, and cook for 20 minutes.

▶ Grind the spices in a mortar or coffee grinder and add them to the vegetables along with the cabbage, water, and tomatoes. Raise the heat and bring the tagine to a boil. Reduce the heat to low, add tempeh, and simmer, uncovered, for 20 to 30 minutes or until the vegetables are tender and the tagine has thickened.

▶ Adjust the seasonings with salt or squeeze of lemon juice to taste. Serve over couscous or rice and sprinkle with cilantro, parsley or chives.

Servings: 8

Mushroom & Garlic Broth

This is a very healing soup that I love to make when I need an immune booster. It's loaded with garlic and mushrooms which have vitality building properties. Shiitake mushrooms are high in iron and a good source of protein. They have been shown to contain many health-promoting compounds that work to stimulate the immune system, lower cholesterol, improve circulation and life energy. Garlic contains the sulfur compounds which promote antioxidant activity to function as a strong antibacterial and antiviral agent...which means it helps fight viruses! Adding seaweed to the broth is an easy way to increase the mineral and nutrient content of the soup, especially with Iodine, without increasing the calories. I love to make a nice vegetable broth ahead of time and use it in this recipe in place of the commercial broth.

- ½ cup barley
- 2 tablespoons olive oil
- 4 ounces shiitake mushrooms, stemmed and thinly sliced (at least 1 cup)
- 8 ounces button mushrooms, sliced thin
- 10 cloves garlic, peeled and thinly sliced
- ¼ cup brown rice vinegar
- 4 cups low sodium vegetable broth
- 1 strip kombu
- 1 bunch kale, stemmed and chopped

▶ Rinse and soak the barley in a large bowl overnight or for 30 minutes before cooking.

▶ Heat the oil in a saucepan over medium heat. Add the mushrooms, and season with sea salt, if desired. Sauté mushrooms for about 10 minutes, or until they begin to brown. Add the garlic, and sauté 2 more minutes. Stir in the vinegar and simmer until it is almost evaporated. Stir to scrape up the brown bits from the pan.

▶ Drain the barley and add to the mushrooms along with the broth, 1 cup of water, and the seaweed. Bring to a boil, then reduce heat to medium-low, and simmer 20 minutes. Add the kale, and cook another 10 to 20 minutes, until kale is tender. Season with salt and pepper. Remove kombu strip.

▶ Serve warm, topped with a dash of tamari and a sprinkle of sesame seeds.

Servings: 8

MUSHROOM SAUCE OR STEW

Another mushroom dish that tastes delicious served over mashed root vegetables, mashed potatoes, polenta, or any kind of burger. Sometimes I use it as a sauce and other times it becomes a nice stew.

- ¼ cup olive oil
- 1 large onion, chopped
- 2 teaspoons fresh rosemary, minced
- Sea salt and freshly ground pepper
- 2 pinches red pepper flakes
- ¼ pound Portobello mushrooms, chopped
- ½ pound white mushrooms, (about 16 ounces), sliced

- 3 ounces shiitake mushrooms, chopped
- 1 leek, white only, chopped
- 2 cloves garlic, minced
- 2 tablespoons tomato paste
- 1 cup vegetable or mushroom stock
- 2 tablespoons fresh parsley, chopped
- 1 tablespoon red wine vinegar

▶ Heat 1 tablespoon of the oil in a large skillet over medium heat. Add the onion and leeks and cook, stirring occasionally, until browned, about 12 minutes. Season with salt and pepper and red pepper flakes and remove to a bowl.

▶ Return the pan to medium heat and add half the remaining oil. When it's hot, add the Portobello mushrooms and sauté until nicely browned, about 5 minutes. Add them to the onion and repeat with the remaining oil and white and shiitake mushrooms.

▶ Return everything to the pan and add the garlic, tomato paste, stock, and vinegar. Simmer gently for 12 to 15 minutes. Add the parsley, taste for salt and pepper.

Servings: 8

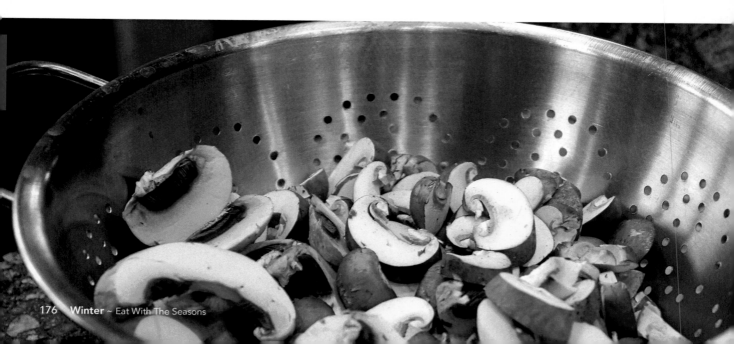

SPICY MOROCCAN CHICKPEAS

This recipe is a little different than my normal repertoire but I like it because it has a nice combination of sweet and spicy and is very warming for a cold winter evening. Although there are many ingredients, there are only two steps to the recipe.

- ¼ cup extra virgin olive oil
- 3 large garlic cloves, peeled
- 2 cups red onion, thinly sliced
- ½ cup dried apricots, thinly sliced
- 1 tablespoon garam masala
- 1 teaspoon sea salt
- ¾ teaspoon black pepper freshly ground
- ¼ teaspoon red pepper flakes
- 1, 3-inch cinnamon stick
- ½ cup water
- 1½ teaspoon grated lemon rind

- 1½ tablespoon fresh lemon juice
- 4 cups cooked chickpeas (or use canned organic chickpeas, drained)
- 1 can (28-ounce) whole tomatoes, drained and chopped
- 6 cups escarole (or use spinach or kale), shredded by hand
- 1 cup cilantro, chopped
- ¼ cup mint springs
- ½ cup almonds, toasted, and chopped
- 4 cups hot whole wheat couscous

▶ Heat a large skillet over medium heat. Add oil to the pan and swirl to coat. Add garlic, cook for 1 minute stirring constantly. Remove garlic from the pan using a slotted spoon; discard. Add onion and next 6 ingredients (through cinnamon stick) to pan; sauté for 7 minutes or until the onion is lightly browned, stirring occasionally. Add ½ cup water, rind, juice, chickpeas, and tomatoes; bring to a boil. Reduce heat, and simmer for 7 minutes, stirring occasionally.

▶ Stir in escarole, (or other greens); simmer for 1 minute or until escarole wilts. Remove from heat. Sprinkle with cilantro and mint; top with almonds. Serve over couscous.

Servings: 8

Sweet Carrots

Great for that winter sweet tooth!

- 4 cups carrots, diagonally sliced
- 1 tablespoon sunflower or olive oil
- ½ teaspoon mustard seeds
- ½ teaspoon turmeric
- ½ teaspoon sea salt
- 1 teaspoon coriander powder
- 1 jalapeño chile pepper, seeded and minced
- 3 tablespoons water or broth
- 1 teaspoon maple syrup

▶ Wash and slice carrots. In a heavy skillet heat the oil and add mustard seeds. When they pop, add turmeric, carrots, coriander, and pepper. Cook uncovered over medium heat, stirring frequently for 2 to 3 minutes. Add water and maple syrup; cover and cook for 5 minutes more over low heat.

Servings: 6

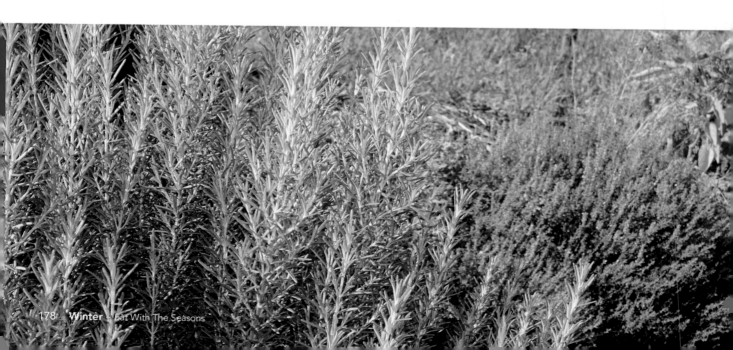

WARM SESAME GREENS MIX

This is another version of leafy greens that enhances any main dish and brings much needed phytonutrients to the plate.

- 1 tablespoon toasted sesame seeds
- 2 tablespoons tamari
- 1 tablespoon rice vinegar
- 2 tablespoons extra virgin olive oil
- 3 garlic cloves, minced
- 1 teaspoon fresh ginger (or to taste), minced
- 5 cups mixed greens, chopped spinach, Swiss chard, bok choy, kale, collards
- 2 teaspoons dark sesame oil

▶ Combine first 4 ingredients in a small bowl, stirring with a whisk.

▶ Heat 1 tablespoon of the olive oil in a large Dutch oven or large skillet over medium heat. Add garlic and ginger, and cook for 1 minute, stirring frequently. Gradually add tougher greens first (collards, kale) with about ¼ cup water, cover and let cook for about 8 minutes. Once they are wilted add the lighter greens (bok choy, Swiss chard, spinach), stirring to mix, and let those wilt also, cooking for about 4 more minutes.

▶ Remove cover and let water evaporate, adding in 1 tablespoon olive oil and mixing. Let the greens finish cooking. Drizzle the sesame oil over the greens.

▶ Drizzle the tamari mixture over the greens and toss well so that the dressing is absorbed.

▶ Place greens in a medium bowl, top with extra sesame seeds and serve warm.

Servings: 4

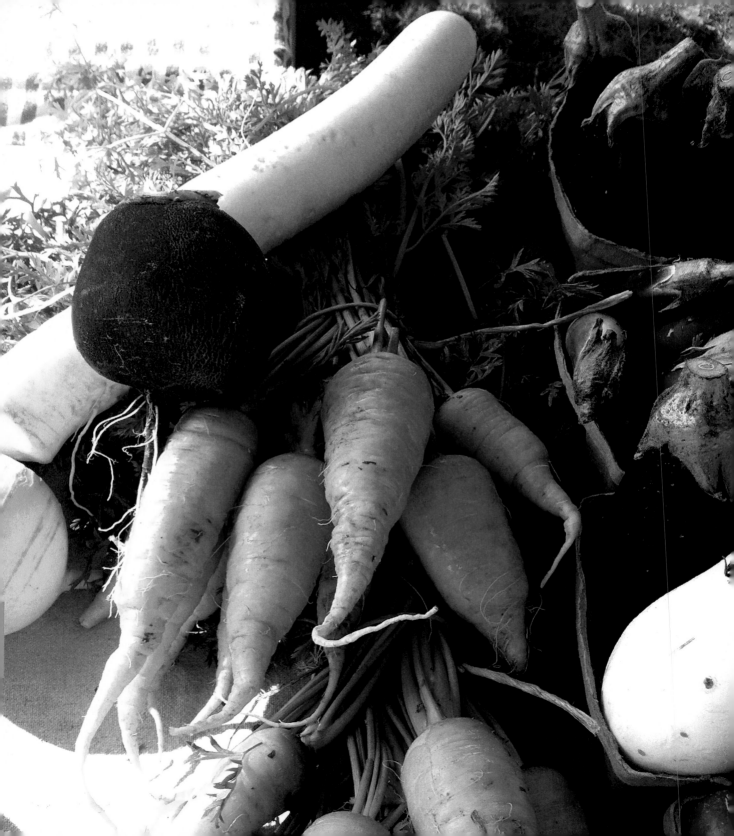

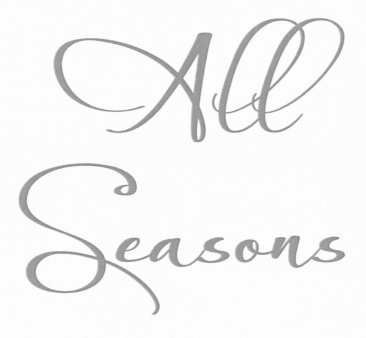

All Seasons

*"To everything there is a season,
A time for every purpose under the sun,
A time to be born and a time to die,
A time to plant and a time to
pluck up that which is planted."*
— Ecclesiastes 3:1-4

Herbs For All Seasons

Culinary Herbs... What do I do with them?

BASIL
- An annual with mild flavor. Easy to grow from seed
- Able to freeze whole leaves or combine with garlic and olive oil in food processor then freeze
- *Tastes Good With:* many vegetables (especially tomatoes), oils, pesto, sauces, chicken and fish, crust, butters and, cheeses

HERBES DE PROVENÇE
- Includes marjoram, thyme, rosemary, savory, tarragon, lavender
- *Tastes Good With:* soups, stews, roasted veggies, roasts and chicken

ROSEMARY
- A robust flavor. Tender perennial, medicinal
- *Tastes Good With:* lamb, chicken, fish, potatoes, and bean dishes

PARSLEY
- A biennial with a mild taste and easy to use with a variety of dishes. Also medicinal and very high in phytonutrients
- *Tastes Good With:* vegetables, grains, beans, broths, soups and stews, salads and pistou

SAGE
- A perennial with a robust flavor
- Medicinal for digestive issues, anti-viral
- *Tastes Good With:* turkey, liver, pork, goat cheese and tea

BAY
- A tender perennial with a mild taste
- *Tastes Good With:* chowders, vegetables, tomato sauces, poultry, fish and stock

CILANTRO (CORIANDER), CHINESE OR MEXICAN PARSLEY
- An annual with mild flavor
- Used for medicinal purposes in India and China. Has detoxifying qualities
- *Tastes Good With:* garlic, citrus, spicy foods, salsas, grains, bean salads, fish and avocados

TARRAGON
- Very strong flavor that can overpower dishes. Tender perennial
- *Tastes Good With:* chicken, fish, eggs and in vinegars

BOUQUET GARNI
- Traditionally made with thyme, bay, parsley tied together in a bundle
- *Add To:* soups, stocks, stews, beans/legumes and poultry

THYME
- A tender perennial with a robust flavor
- Anti-viral, anti microbial medicinal uses
- *Tastes Good With:* tomatoes and other vegetables, olives, poultry, roasts, soups and stews and mushrooms

DILL
- Annual with mild taste. Seeds very easily.
- *Tastes Good With:* early summer vegetables (leeks, cucumber, etc.), yogurt sauce, fish, vinegar, breads/crackers and eggs

LAVENDER
- A perennial with many varieties adapting to climate. A mild taste
- Medicinal uses for stress and relaxation among a few: use essential oils
- *Tastes Good With:* sweets (ice creams, jam, honey, etc.) and beverages

CUMIN
- Originates in Middle East and India
- An annual
- Medicinal uses (Sudan- Asia): indigestion and stimulant
- *Tastes Good With:* chili powder, stews, lentils and toast

CARAWAY
- A tropical perennial
- Medicinal uses: anti-viral
- *Tastes Good With:* fruit, sauces, salsas, spice blends, soups and stews, sauerkraut, bread

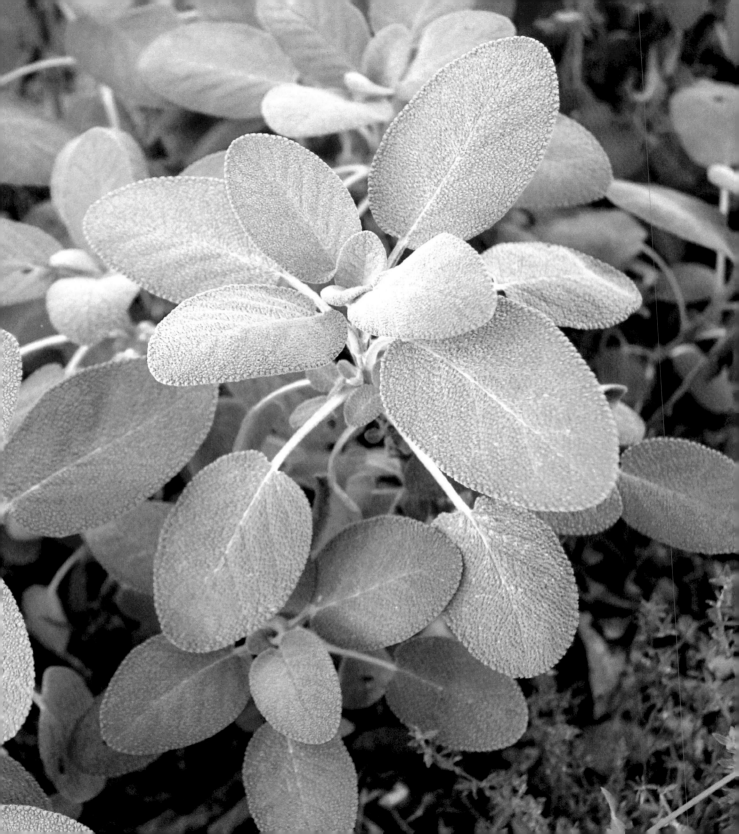

Dips, Sauces & Marinades

BASIL OIL

This is the easiest oil to make and it tastes so great drizzled over just about anything!

- 2 cups basil leaves, firmly packed
- 1⅓ cup extra virgin olive oil
- Pinch sea salt

▶ Coarsely chop the basil and place into a clean glass jar.

▶ Add a pinch of sea salt and pour olive oil to fill the jar to the brim making sure to stir the basil so that the olive oil covers the basil completely.

▶ Put the lid firmly on the jar and let sit overnight or for a couple of days (at the most), shaking every once in a while.

▶ When you are ready, strain the basil leaves through a tight mesh strainer or a double layer of cheesecloth. Pour back into the jar. Discard the solids or use right away in a soup or other dish.

▶ To strain even further you may put it through a coffee filter. The oil is ready to use and will keep for a week or two in the refrigerator.

Servings: 48 / Yield: 1½ cups

BEAN-GARLIC SPREAD

Great with crudités or pita chips! Or use as a spread on sandwiches in place of mayo.

- 2 cups cannellini or butter beans, rinsed and drained
- ⅓ cup fresh parsley, leaves only
- ⅓ cup water
- 1 tablespoon fresh lemon juice
- 1 tablespoon extra virgin olive oil
- 2 teaspoon roasted garlic paste, or garlic powder, or 1 head of roasted garlic
- ½ teaspoon sea salt, or to taste
- ¼ teaspoon freshly ground pepper
- ¼ teaspoon hot sauce, to taste (if desired, you can also use red pepper flakes)

▶ Place beans and remaining ingredients in a food processor; process until smooth. Let flavors mingle for 1 hour or so before serving.

▶ Can be made 1 or 2 days ahead.

Servings: 8 / Yield: 24 tablespoons

CILANTRO SAUCE

Great condiment for a multitude of uses, from burgers to dip.

- 2 tablespoons fresh lemon juice
- ¼ cup coconut milk (in the can)
- ½ - to 1whole jalapeño chile pepper, seeded and minced
- 1 clove garlic
- 1, 1-inch piece fresh ginger, peeled and minced
- ¼ teaspoon sea salt
- 1 cup cilantro (or mint)

▶ Combine lemon juice, coconut milk, chile, garlic, ginger, salt, and cilantro in a blender or food processor and blend until smooth.

Servings: 4

FETA DILL DRESSING

I got this recipe from The Whole Foods Cookbook. I like this dressing when I have a simple salad that needs a little lift. It pairs really well with cucumbers.

- 1 cup yogurt
- 3 tablespoons finely crumbled feta cheese
- 1 tablespoon lemon juice
- 1 tablespoon minced fresh dill
- 2 teaspoons lemon pepper

▶ Combine the yogurt, feta cheese, lemon juice, dill, and lemon pepper in a large bowl or blender. Refrigerate.

Servings: 12 / Yield: 1¼ cups

Harissa

A little bit of this spicy condiment goes a long way to give soups, stews and grains and beans a zip! The aroma from the spices is so intense. This will keep for quite while in the refrigerator.

- 2 teaspoons whole cumin seeds
- 1 teaspoon whole caraway seeds
- 2½ tablespoons extra virgin olive oil
- 4 teaspoons freshly squeezed lemon juice
- 2 teaspoons ground cayenne pepper
- Pinch of sea salt

▶ In a mortar or clean coffee mill, grind the cumin, caraway, and salt to a powder.

▶ Transfer the ground spices to a bowl if you are using the coffee mill.

▶ Stir in the olive oil, lemon juice, and cayenne.

Servings: 8 / Yield: ¼ cup

Herbed Tofu-Yogurt Sour Cream

One of my all-time favorite sauces that I love to use on burgers, vegetables and as a dip. It pairs especially well with beans. This is my substitute for sour cream.

- 4 tablespoon fresh lemon juice
- 4 tablespoon fresh lime juice (optional)
- ½ pound firm tofu
- 1 cup plain yogurt
- 2 teaspoons Dijon style mustard
- ⅓ cup extra-virgin olive oil
- ½ cup chopped cilantro
- ¼ cup chopped parsley
- ¼ cup mixed herbs like rosemary, chives, tarragon, oregano, optional
- 1 teaspoon sea salt
- 1 teaspoon tamari
- Pinch cayenne pepper
- 1 garlic clove, pressed, or to taste
- 1 scallion, thinly sliced (optional)

▶ Put all ingredients in blender and blend until smooth.

▶ Let sit for an hour or so to let the flavors blend. The sour cream will keep in the refrigerator for up to 3 days.

Servings: 24

Homemade Mayonnaise (Aioli)

So good with fish!! This is easy to make and much better quality than the mayonnaise that you buy commercially. You can adjust the garlic to your liking.

- 1 egg, organic or free range
- 1 tablespoon mustard, like Dijon or whole grain (optional)
- ¾ teaspoon sea salt
- 2 tablespoons fresh lemon juice
- 1 cup extra virgin olive oil
- 1 to 2 cloves garlic

▶ In a blender, combine the egg, mustard, salt, lemon juice, and garlic. Blend for 30 seconds or until completely mixed.

▶ With the blender running on low speed, add the oil very, slowly in a very thin stream, until the mixture has emulsified and becomes thick like mayonnaise. The last ⅓ cup may be added a little faster if you see that the oil is absorbing well. Taste and adjust the seasonings. Transfer to a jar and refrigerate until ready to use.

Servings: 8 / Yield: 1 cup

Hummus

An easy snack that I use as a spread instead of mayo, as well as a dip.

- 2 cans (15-ounce each) chickpeas, drained and rinsed
- 2 large garlic cloves
- 4 to 6 tablespoons fresh lemon juice
- 2 tablespoons olive oil
- 3 tablespoons tahini
- ½ teaspoon ground cumin
- 1 teaspoon sea salt, (to taste)
- ½ cup low-fat plain yogurt

▶ Drain the beans and puree along with the garlic in a food processor or blender. Add the lemon juice, olive oil, tahini, cumin, salt to taste, and yogurt and blend until thoroughly smooth. Taste and adjust seasonings, adding more salt, garlic, or lemon juice as needed.

▶ Transfer to a serving bowl and cover. Refrigerate until ready to serve. Will keep for about 5 days.

Servings: 12

Hummus-Parsley Dip

Hummus is one of those snacks that I feel really good eating because it has lots of protein and fiber but minimal fat. It can be eaten with vegetables or crackers, on a sandwich in place of mayo, or just with a spoon! This version of the basic recipe includes parsley but it could just as well be cilantro.

- 1 clove garlic
- ½ cup fresh parsley leaves (or cilantro)
- 1 can (15-ounce) chickpeas, rinsed and drained
- ¼ cup Greek yogurt
- 3 tablespoons tahini

- 2 tablespoons toasted sesame oil
- 1½ teaspoon grated lemon peel
- 1½ teaspoon ground cumin
- 1 teaspoon sea salt, to taste
- ¼ teaspoon cayenne pepper

▶ In a food processor coarsely chop garlic and parsley. Add beans and blend 30 seconds. Add remaining ingredients and blend until smooth.

▶ Serve with pita chips, raw vegetables or use as a spread in sandwiches.

Servings: 20

Marinade for Chicken or Salmon

This is especially good on my wild-caught Alaskan salmon that is brought to us from a young couple who goes out to Alaska each year to fish. They bring it back to us flash-frozen so we can enjoy the most delicious fish there is.

- ¼ cup olive oil
- 2 tablespoons tamari or shoyu
- 2 tablespoons balsamic vinegar
- 2 tablespoons green onion, finely chopped
- 1 clove garlic, minced

- ¾ teaspoon ground ginger
- 1 teaspoon red pepper flakes
- ½ teaspoon sesame oil
- ¼ teaspoon sea salt

▶ Place fish or chicken in a medium, non-porous glass dish. In a separate bowl, combine all the ingredients for the marinade and whisk together.

▶ Pour over fish or chicken. If using fish, cover and marinate no more than 1 hour. If using chiken, cover and marinate for at least 4 hours or overnight.

▶ You can cook your fish on an outdoor grill, or broil in the oven until the fish flakes with a fork.

▶ For chicken you can bake in the oven, cook in parchment, or sauté in a pan with other vegetables.

Servings: 6

Roasted Garlic, Sun-Dried Tomato & White Bean Dip

This is an easy, quick recipe for healthy entertaining.

- 1 head garlic, with loose paper removed
- 1 cup water
- 4 ounces sun-dried tomatoes* in oil; drained, oil reserved, chopped,
  or use dried sun-dried tomatoes and follow recipe for soaking
- 2 tablespoons extra virgin olive oil
- ½ teaspoon fresh rosemary, finely chopped
- ¼ teaspoon sea salt
- ¼ teaspoon freshly ground black pepper
- 1 can (15-ounce) organic great northern beans, rinsed and drained
- ½ lemon, freshly squeezed (or to taste)

▶ Preheat oven to 375°F.

▶ Remove white papery skin from garlic head but do not peel off cloves. Put in foil and drizzle with about 1 teaspoon of olive oil. Wrap up and bake for about 45 minutes; cool for 10 minutes. Separate cloves; squeeze to extract garlic pulp. Discard skins.

▶ If using sun-dried tomatoes that are not in olive oil; bring 1 cup water to a boil in a saucepan, add tomatoes, cover and remove from heat. Let stand 10 minutes. Drain tomatoes in a colander over a bowl and reserve ¼ cup of the liquid. Chop.

▶ If you are using sun-dried tomatoes in olive oil, chop tomatoes and set aside.

▶ Place garlic pulp, tomatoes, ¼ cup reserved liquid, olive oil, beans and salt and pepper, in a food processor; process until smooth.

Servings: 15

SOY & ROASTED GARLIC DRESSING

Roasted garlic gives this Asian-inspired dressing a deep, nutty flavor. It's great on any combination of salad greens, cooked leafy greens, or use it as a dipping sauce.

- 1 head garlic
- 4 tablespoons extra virgin olive oil
- Juice of 1 lime
- 2 tablespoons red-wine vinegar

- 1 tablespoon grated fresh ginger
- 1 tablespoon toasted sesame oil
- 1 tablespoon reduced-sodium soy sauce or tamari
- Freshly ground black pepper to taste

▶ Preheat oven to 400°F.

▶ Rub excess papery skin off garlic head without separating cloves. Slice the tip off, exposing the ends of the cloves. Place the garlic head on a piece of foil, drizzle with 1 tablespoon olive oil and wrap into a package. Put in a baking dish and bake until the garlic is very soft, 40 minutes to 1 hour. Unwrap and let cool slightly.

▶ Squeeze the garlic pulp into a blender or food processor (discard the skins). Add the remaining 3 tablespoons olive oil, lime juice, vinegar, ginger, sesame oil and soy sauce; blend or process until smooth. Season with pepper.

Servings: 10

TAPENADE

I love the flexibility of tapenade. This is a staple in our house. I use it as a spread for appetizers, a condiment on fish or chicken, and to flavor pizza and polenta. It adds such a nice salty flavor.

- ½ pound black Greek olives, pitted (1⅓ cups)
- 2 large garlic cloves
- 1½ tablespoon drained capers
- 4 to 6 anchovies to taste
- ½ to 1 teaspoon fresh thyme (or ½ teaspoon dried)
- ½ to 1 teaspoon fresh rosemary (for dried use ¼ teaspoon crushed)

- 2 tablespoons lemon juice
- 1 teaspoon Dijon style mustard
- 2 tablespoons extra virgin olive oil
- Lots of freshly ground pepper
- 1 to 2 tablespoon Cognac (optional)

▶ Pit the olives and puree along with the garlic, capers, anchovies, thyme, and rosemary in a mortar and pestle or food processor. Add the remaining ingredients and continue to process until you have a smooth paste. Place in a bowl, cover, and refrigerate until ready to use.

Servings: 24

Mustard Vinaigrette Dressing

This is my all time favorite dressing for salads. It's what I grew up on. It's very easy to make and you can adjust the quantity based on how much you need. I like to make extra so that I have enough to last for a few days of salads.

- 3 to 4 tablespoons lemon juice (or you can substitute apple cider or red wine vinegar if desired)
- 2 teaspoons Dijon mustard
- 1 teaspoon garlic powder, or
  1 clove pressed garlic (optional),
- Sea salt and freshly ground pepper to taste.
- 6 to 7 tablespoons extra virgin olive oil

▶ In a small bowl, blend with a whisk, lemon juice (or vinegar), with Dijon mustard.

▶ Add garlic powder or minced garlic (optional), sea salt and freshly ground pepper to taste.

▶ Add in 6 to 7 tablespoons good quality, extra virgin olive oil and mix very well so that ingredients thicken and blend completely. Use an immersion blender or mixer if desired.

▶ Add minced herbs if desired.

Servings: 10

Yogurt Tahini Sauce

- ½ cup low fat plain yogurt
- 2 tablespoons tahini
- 1 tablespoon fresh lemon juice
- ½ cup fresh parsley leaves, chopped
- 1 clove fresh garlic, minced or added to blender (optional)
- ¼ teaspoon salt

▶ Combine yogurt, tahini, lemon juice, parsley and salt in a bowl or blender until well blended.

Servings: 12 / Yield: 24 tablespoons

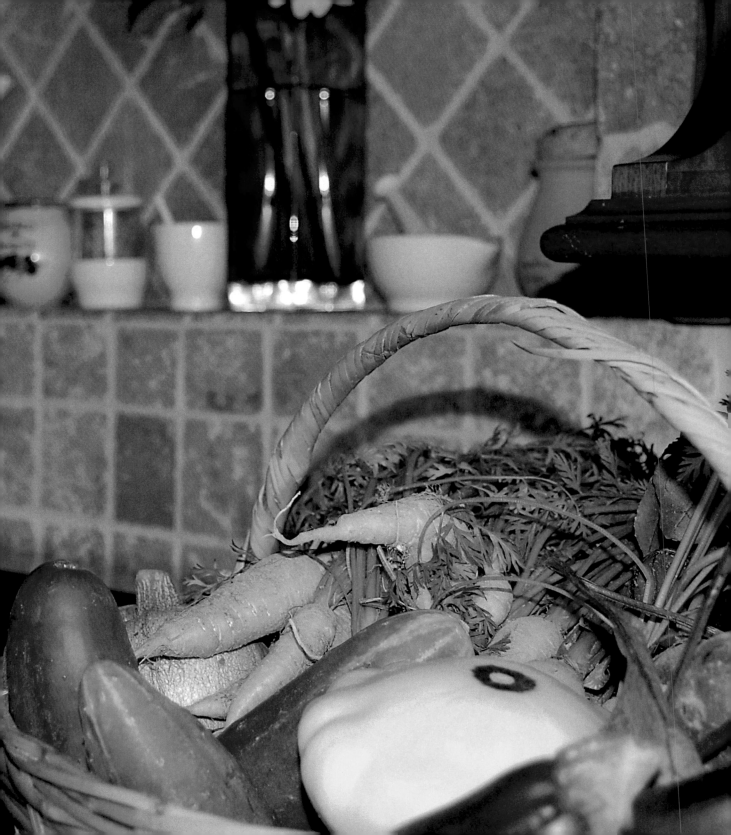

?

What's for
Dinner

Under-30-Minute Menu Ideas

In my experience raising children and having a very hectic household, these are some of the recipes that used to work for us. They were tried and true and the children would eat them, no questions asked. They can work for any household on the go.

Frozen chicken cutlets in parchment with spinach, lemon, (use other veggies on hand), some type of quick cooking grain like quinoa or whole wheat couscous, lettuce mix (from the bag) with cucumbers, olives, cherry tomatoes, feta cheese

Quick tomato soup with rice (or substitute quinoa), grilled Gruyère cheese on whole grain bread, salad

Provençal chicken stew with beans rather than potatoes (use a small pasta), bread, salad

Potato leek soup (with any vegetables you have, like carrots, celery, broccoli, spinach), Make Your Own Humus roll-ups with any veggies you have on hand (sprouts, cucumbers, olives, grated cheese, cherry tomatoes, seeds, lettuce, chicken pieces, ground turkey)

Easy bake quinoa with baby spinach, (or steamed broccoli)

Ragout of chickpeas and tomatoes over whole wheat couscous, salad

Salad of greens, cottage cheese, sunflower seeds, chickpeas, cucumbers, tomatoes, olives and other vegetables that you like, served with pita bread

Omelet with a salad (or in bread as a sandwich)

Breakfast for dinner, creamy oatmeal with raisins, cinnamon and almond milk or spelt pancakes with fruit

Stir fry of chicken cutlets, shrimp, or tofu, vegetables like broccoli, spinach, carrots, mushrooms, served over rice or whole wheat couscous

Cardamom pasta salad, served with sautéed spinach or other greens

Crustless vegetable pie (without the pistou, or using jarred pesto), with a salad

Snappy salmon burgers (using canned salmon), herbed yogurt spread (made with Greek yogurt and your favorite spice blend), baked potato, quick salad or greens

Mediterranean whole wheat pasta salad (or Udon Noodles) made with broccoli, cherry tomatoes, canned tuna, cucumbers, olives, and a mustard vinaigrette

Spinach salad with cranberries, croutons and chicken, page 86. To assemble quickly, substitute a simple mustard vinaigrette dressing in place of the vinaigrette called for in the recipe.

Summer tomato sauce over pasta with a salad

Salad niçoise with whole grain bread

Home version of an Egg McMuffin: make an egg, put it in a whole grain english muffin with cheese, wrap in foil and put in the oven to melt.

Baked potatoes topped with chili and salsa

CARDAMOM PASTA SALAD

This is the easiest salad to make and great to bring to a summer picnic.

- 1 package of udon noodles or whole wheat linguini
- ¼ cup tamari soy sauce
- ¼ cup extra virgin olive oil
- ¼ cup sesame seeds
- 1 teaspoon cardamom
- 3 tablespoons sundried tomatoes, or to taste
- 2 tablespoons scallions
- ¼ teaspoon red pepper flakes
- ¼ cup feta cheese, or more to taste

▶ Boil the water for pasta to cook. Cook as directed and then rinse well under cold water. Sprinkle tamari on pasta and mix well with hands so that the tamari gets absorbed into all the pasta. Add more if desired.

▶ Heat olive oil in a pan and toast sesame seeds until brown. Add the cardamom at the end and mix well.

▶ Pour mixture over pasta and squeeze in with hands.

▶ Cut desired amount of sun-dried tomatoes into small pieces and mix into pasta along with red pepper flakes, to taste. Garnish with scallions and feta cheese. Let sit for at least 20 minutes to let flavors absorb into pasta. Serve at room temperature. Can be chilled in refrigerator for up to 3 days.

Servings: 6

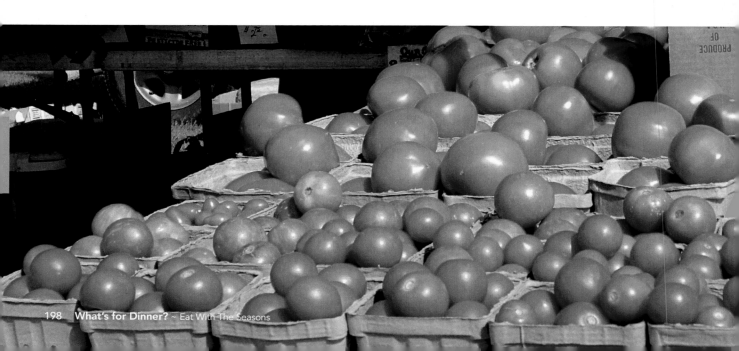

EASY DINNER OMELET

This is the most versatile, easy meal to prepare. We ate this quite a bit for dinner when I was young and I often served it to my family when we were in a rush to get off to practices and events. It tastes great served with whole grain bread and a nice green salad with vinaigrette dressing.

- 2 tablespoons olive oil
- 1 medium potato, peeled and chopped
- 1 small onion, chopped
- 1 clove garlic, minced
- 4 eggs, lightly beaten
- 1 tablespoon basil, parsley or marjoram, chopped
- 2 ounces goat cheese, crumbled
- Sea salt and freshly ground pepper

▶ Heat 1 tablespoon of the oil in a medium non-stick pan and add the potatoes. Stir a bit and then add about ¼ cup of water, cover and cook until done, about 4 minutes, making sure not to burn. Take the cover off and let the water evaporate. Add 1 more tablespoon of oil to the pan and continue to cook the potatoes.

▶ Add the onions to the potatoes and cook until translucent. Add the garlic and stir for about 3 minutes so that all the flavors blend.

▶ Meanwhile, beat the eggs in a bowl with a few pinches of salt and some pepper. Stir in your herb of choice.

▶ Check your pan for oil and be sure there is enough. Carefully pour the eggs over the potato mixture so that it spreads out over the whole skillet. Cook for a minute or so on medium heat and then shuffle the pan or lift the sides of the egg mixture so that the eggs run underneath and cook evenly.

▶ After the omelet is mostly cooked, crumble some goat cheese, or other cheese of choice, over the top.

▶ Continue to cook over medium heat until the eggs are set about 10 minutes or so. Keep an eye on the eggs and keep lifting to make sure they stay loose on the bottom. Then, to melt the cheese and make sure the omelet is cooked on top, you can either cover the top with a lid or foil, or you can slide the pan into the oven if pan is ovenproof. Invert onto a serving platter and serve topped with chopped parsley or basil. Cut into wedges and serve warm.

Servings: 4

EASY QUINOA BAKE

This is a great crowd pleaser and easy to prepare. I call it my mac'n cheese replacement. Also easy to reheat for tomorrow's lunch.

- 1 cup quinoa, rinsed
- 2 cups veggie stock or water
- 4 ounces goat cheese
- 4 ounces Gruyère cheese, grated
- 2 eggs

- 1 bunch chives, chopped
- 2 teaspoons garlic powder (optional)
- 1 tablespoon extra virgin olive oil
- Salt and pepper to taste

▶ Toast quinoa in medium hot pan for about 3 minutes. Add the water or stock and cook until all water is absorbed.

▶ Meanwhile beat eggs. Add cheeses and stir well. Add chives, oil, salt, pepper and garlic powder. Add to quinoa.

▶ Spread quinoa mix into an oiled 8x8-inch baking pan and bake in a 350ºF oven for about 20 minutes. Cut into pieces and serve warm with extra Parmesan grated on top if desired.

Servings: 8

QUICK TOMATO SOUP WITH RICE

This was one of my favorite soups that my mom used to make for us when we were little. She worked all day and would come home and make this soup rather than serve the high sodium canned versions that are out there. I used to love it with a grilled cheese or tuna sandwich.

- 2 tablespoons olive oil
- 1 medium onion, chopped
- 2 cloves garlic, minced
- 1 can (28-ounce) tomatoes, chopped
- 8 cups broth, chicken stock, or water
- 1 bay leaf

- ½ teaspoon dried thyme
- 1 teaspoon marjoram leaves, chopped, or dried marjoram
- ½ cup brown basmati rice, rinsed
- Sea salt and pepper to taste

▶ In a soup pot or Dutch oven, heat the olive oil. Add the onions and sauté for a few minutes until they turn translucent. Add the minced garlic, stir and let cook for another few minutes. Add the chopped tomatoes and all the herbs and stir. Let cook for about 5 minutes.

▶ Pour in the broth and bring to a boil. Turn down to a simmer and add the rice. Cook for about 25 minutes, partially covered, until rice is cooked. Add sea salt and pepper to taste. Serve topped with Parmesan or Romano cheese.

Servings: 8

Ragout of Chickpeas & Tomatoes

This is a very flavorful easy-to-prepare dish. It will last for about a week in the refrigerator. When chopping the jalapeño, be careful not to touch your eyes, or as the purists say, wear gloves.

- 1 tablespoon olive oil
- 1 jalapeño pepper, seeded and cut into ¼-inch squares
- 1 large onion cut into ½-inch pieces
- 3 large garlic cloves, minced
- 1 tablespoon ground cumin
- 2 small zucchini, chopped
- 2 cans (15-ounce each) chickpeas, drained and rinsed
  OR 1 can (16-ounce) black beans, thoroughly rinsed and drained, and 1 can (15-ounce) chickpeas
- 1 can (28-ounce) plum tomatoes, chopped
- ¼ cup parsley chopped
- Juice of 1 lemon or lime
- Salt

▶ Heat the oil in a large saucepan (with a cover) and sauté jalapeno and onion for 4 minutes, stirring frequently.

▶ Add the garlic and sauté 1 minute. Add the cumin and zucchini and sauté 5 minutes. Add the beans and tomatoes, cover and simmer for 10 minutes, stirring several times. Add the parsley, lemon juice and salt to taste.

▶ Serve hot.

Servings: 8

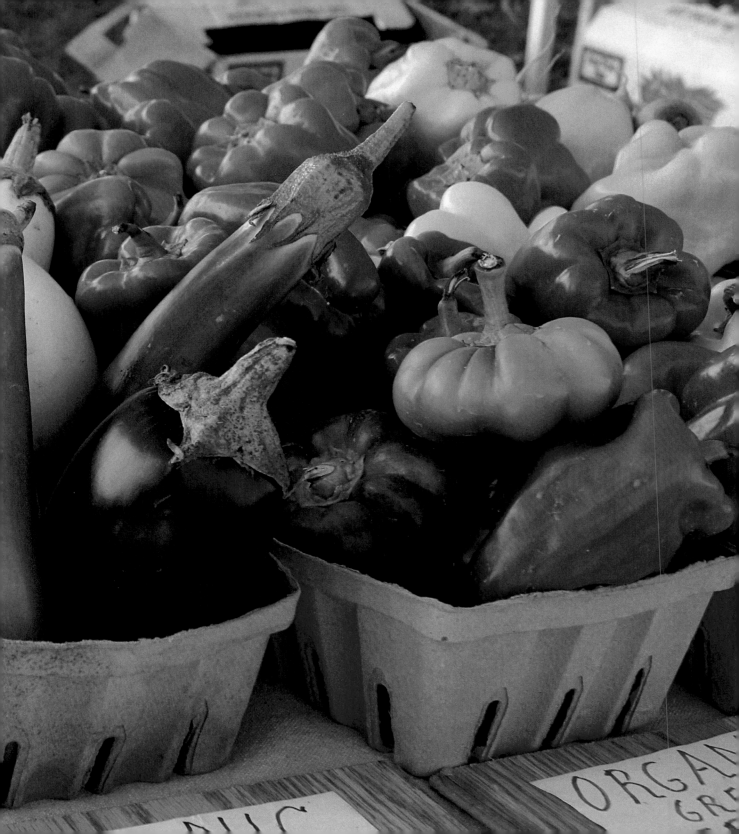

Other Recipes

These recipes are perfect anytime of year.

Black Bean Burgers

This recipe seems rather labor intensive but I included it because it makes quite a few patties and I like to freeze them in little baggies after I cook them and take them out for a quick meal.

- 4 cups black beans
- 1 cup peeled and diced (or grated) carrots, sautéed
- 1 cup peeled and diced onion, sautéed
- 1 clove garlic, minced
- ¾ cup diced red bell pepper (optional)
- ¾ cup diced green or yellow bell pepper (optional)
- ½ teaspoon sea salt
- ½ cup plus 1 teaspoon extra-virgin olive oil
- ¾ cup cornmeal
- ½ teaspoon ground cumin
- 2 tablespoons chili powder
- ¼ teaspoon cayenne
- 1 cup chickpea flour
- 3 teaspoons fresh lemon juice
- ½ cup chopped cilantro or parsley
- 8 whole wheat buns
- Sliced tomatoes, for garnish
- Lettuce, for garnish

▶ In a large saucepan, simmer the beans in 5 cups of water for 35 minutes or until tender. Drain the beans, reserving 1 cup of the cooking liquid.

▶ Sauté onions, carrots, garlic, peppers over medium heat for 5 minutes or so.

▶ In a large bowl, mix together the carrots, onion, peppers (optional), salt, 1 teaspoon olive oil, and cornmeal. Stir in the cumin, chili powder, cayenne, chickpea flour, lemon juice, and cilantro. Stir in the black beans and form into patties. Add a bit of the reserved cooking liquid to the mixture to moisten if it is too dry. Or if you prefer a smoother-textured burger, blend half of the mixture in a blender until smooth and combine with the remaining mixture.

▶ In a skillet, heat the remaining ½ cup olive oil and cook the burgers for about 2 minutes on each side. Or, bake in a 325°F oven on a cookie sheet sprinkled with corn meal, for about 15 minutes. Serve on whole wheat buns with a slice of tomato, lettuce, and avocado. Or serve without rolls and with a mango salsa or herbed garlic spread.

Servings: 8

Brown Rice & Lentil Burgers

I learned this recipe from my sister who has been a vegetarian since way back. She always recommends the most delicious combinations and this is one of them. When I plan my meals I like to arrange it so I have leftover rice and lentils to make these patties later in the week. They taste delicious topped with herbed yogurt sauce.

- ½ cup lentils, rinsed
- 1 pound mushrooms, chopped
- 1 cup brown rice
- 1 teaspoon sea salt
- 2 tablespoons extra virgin olive oil
- 1 teaspoon chili powder
- 2 cloves garlic, chopped
- 1 medium red onion, chopped
- ¼ cup bread crumbs
- 1 egg slightly beaten

▶ In a medium saucepan, bring 1½ cups of water to a boil. Add the lentils, reduce heat, and cook until softened, about 15 minutes. Drain and set aside.

▶ Meanwhile, in another medium saucepan, bring 2 cups of water to a boil, add the rice, reduce the heat, cover, and simmer until the rice is just tender, about 40 minutes. Drain and set aside.

▶ In a sauté pan, heat the olive oil over medium heat and sauté the onions until translucent. Add the garlic and mushrooms and sauté until juice flows from mushrooms, about 4 minutes.

▶ Preheat oven to 350°F.

▶ In a large bowl, combine the lentils, rice and vegetables. Add the salt and chili powder and mix well. Add a bit of breadcrumbs to hold the mixture together, if needed. You can also add an egg to hold it together. Make into burger-sized patties and place on a baking pan, or press into a loaf pan. Bake burgers until slightly firm, about 15 minutes, or bake the loaf for about 25 minutes. You can also cook the patties in a skillet with olive oil.

Servings: 8

Chicken Stew Provençal

Probably my all time favorite chicken stew recipe. I used to make this for the kids all the time when I needed an easy stew. I love the flavor of the fennel and the saffron together along with the garlic. The broth is so delicious! I can eat this anytime of year.

- 6 to 8 chicken thighs, or 1 whole chicken cut into pieces
- 2 tablespoon extra virgin olive oil
- 1 large onion, chopped
- 1 leek, white part only, cleaned and sliced
- 2 large garlic cloves, minced or put through a press
- 1 pound tomatoes, or 1 can (14-ounce) Italian plum tomatoes, diced
- 2 additional garlic cloves, minced
- Sea salt
- 1½ cups white wine

- 2 cups chicken stock
- 1 bay leaf
- ½ teaspoon thyme, more to taste
- ¼ teaspoon fennel seed, crushed
- 2 pinches saffron
- 1 small can white northern beans, (optional), drained and rinsed
- Pinch cayenne pepper
- ¾ pound Yukon Gold potato, peeled and diced
- Freshly ground pepper
- Gruyère or Parmesan cheese, and parsley for garnish

▶ Remove skin from chicken thighs.

▶ Heat olive oil in a large Dutch oven, add chicken pieces and brown on each side, cooking for about 5 minutes. Remove chicken pieces and set aside for later.

▶ To the same pot add a little more olive oil, scraping the bottom to remove any excess chicken, and sauté the onion, leek, and 2 large garlic cloves over low heat for about 10 minutes, stirring to prevent browning.

▶ Add the tomatoes and additional garlic and continue to sauté over medium heat for 5 minutes. Raise the heat and cook over high heat for a few minutes more, stirring.

▶ Add the chicken, salt lightly, and stir together with the tomatoes and onions. Cover and cook about 7 minutes over medium heat, turning the pieces to cook.

▶ Add the wine and bring to a boil. Boil for about 3 minutes then add chicken stock, bay leaf, thyme, fennel seed, saffron, orange peel, and more salt to taste. Bring to a simmer, cover and simmer slowly for about 20 minutes or until chicken is cooked through.

▶ Meanwhile, steam or boil the potatoes and set aside.

▶ When the chicken is almost done, add the beans, if you are using them, and the potatoes. Remove the bay leaf and add just a hint of cayenne, just enough to lift up the flavor of the stew and not overpower it. Add pepper to taste. Garnish with Parmesan cheese and chopped fresh parsley and serve in wide soup bowls.

▶ This will hold for a few days in the refrigerator.

Servings: 6

CHICKPEA PATTIES

These patties are the easiest of all and taste great with any of the salsas or sauces. It makes enough for a crowd (or to freeze for other meals).

- 1 tablespoons extra virgin olive oil
- 1 red onion, finely chopped
- 2 cloves garlic, crushed or pressed
- 1 tablespoon ground cumin
- 2 cans (10-ounce each) chickpeas, drained or 3 cups cooked chickpeas

- ¼ cup sunflower seeds (optional)
- ½ cup finely chopped cilantro
- 2 eggs, lightly beaten
- ⅔ cup chickpea flour

▶ Heat olive oil in a frying pan, add onion and cook over medium heat for 3 minutes or until soft. Add garlic and cumin and cook 1 minute. Remove from heat and cool slightly.

▶ Blend chickpeas, sunflower seeds, cilantro, eggs, and onion mixture in food processor until smooth. Fold in flour and season.

▶ Divide mixture into eight portions and, using floured hands, form into patties.

▶ Heat olive oil in frying pan and cook patties in two batches over medium heat for 2 to 3 minutes on each side, or until firm. Drain. Keep warm.

Servings: 4

CORN BREAD

This comes from an old Yankee Cookbook that I was given when we got married. I have substituted spelt flour for white flour and I love the flavor it brings.

- ¾ cup yellow cornmeal
- 1 cup spelt flour
- 2 teaspoons baking powder
- ½ teaspoon baking soda
- ¾ teaspoon sea salt

- ¼ cup maple syrup
- 1 cup buttermilk, or plain kefir or plain yogurt
- ½ cup milk or almond milk
- 1 egg, lightly beaten
- 2 tablespoons butter, melted*

▶ Preheat the oven to 375°F.

▶ Place all the dry ingredients in a bowl and mix with a wire whisk.

▶ Add the wet ingredients to the dry and mix until blended. Do not over mix. Pour the batter into a greased 9x9-inch pan and bake for 25 minutes.

*If you substitute coconut oil for the butter, it gives a nice nutty flavor.

Servings: 12

CILANTRO-LIME RICE

An easy stir-in of cilantro and lime juice can transform plain cooked rice into a much livelier side dish that's an ideal accompaniment for so many of my main meals, stews, and bean burgers.

- 1 cup long-grain brown rice, or basmati rice
- Coarse salt
- ½ cup fresh cilantro chopped (or a mix of herbs)
- 2 tablespoons fresh lime juice

- 1 tablespoon olive oil
- 1 garlic clove
- Grated Parmesan cheese (optional)

▶ In a medium saucepan, bring 1½ cups water to a boil. Add rice and ¼ teaspoon salt; cover, and reduce to a simmer. cook until water is absorbed and rice is just tender, 16 to 18 minutes.

▶ Meanwhile, in a blender, combine cilantro, lime juice, oil, garlic, and 2 tablespoons water; blend until smooth. Stir into cooked rice, and fluff with a fork.

Servings: 4

FISH (OR CHICKEN) IN PARCHMENT

An easy recipe for days when you are in a hurry to get something healthy on the table. It can work for any season depending on which vegetables you put in with the fish or chicken. You can even do a "build your own" so that everyone can personalize their meal. It does not have to be complicated...just adding a little lemon, spinach, and herb blend can work just as well.

- 3 limes, juiced (or lemons)
- 4 cloves garlic, minced
- 2 mild chili peppers, seeded and sliced
- 1 medium red onion, diced
- 1 strip fresh ginger (or to taste), minced
- ¼ cup olive oil
- 4 heads baby bok choy, rinsed and trimmed
- 4 fillets fish, like cod, halibut, black bass, striped bass, haddock
- 4 cups spinach, stemmed and coarsely chopped, or baby spinach
- ¼ cup cilantro, chopped
- Sea salt and pepper to taste

▶ Preheat oven to 450°F.

▶ In a bowl mix the first five ingredients and the olive oil until blended.

▶ Fold the parchment paper in half and open up. Place baby bok choy on the bottom (on the crease), then place fish on top and any other vegetables that you might be adding to your fillet, like the spinach. Top with the liquid mixture and cilantro, and salt and pepper to taste. Fold up the parchment and seal with a paperclip.

▶ Place parchment packs on a baking sheet and in the oven for about 10 to 12 minutes until fish is just cooked through. (Note: this time is for fish that is about ½-inch thick. If your fish is thinner cook for less time.) Remove packets from the oven — open carefully to let the steam escape — and transfer to serving plates. Serve with rice, couscous, or quinoa.

Servings: 4

GREEK BISON BURGERS

These are one of my favorite burgers because the flavor is all there and it really doesn't need a roll if you don't want the extra bulk (or calories). Bison or grassfed beef are a much more sustainable source of red meat than the corn fed beef that is typically sold.

- 1 pound bison, ground
- ½ cup spinach, cooked and squeezed dry
- ½ cup feta cheese (preferably sheep's-milk), crumbled
- 2 teaspoons fresh dill, chopped
- 1 teaspoon fresh oregano, chopped
- 1 teaspoon cumin, ground
- 1 teaspoon garlic, minced
- ¾ teaspoon kosher salt
- ½ teaspoon freshly ground pepper

▶ Preheat grill to medium-high.

▶ Place bison, spinach, feta, 2 teaspoons dill, oregano, cumin, garlic, ¾ teaspoon salt and ½ teaspoon pepper in a large mixing bowl. Gently combine without over mixing. Form into 4 oval-shaped patties roughly the size of the rolls.

▶ Oil the grill rack. Grill the burgers until an instant-read thermometer inserted into the center registers 155°F, 5 to 6 minutes per side.

▶ Assemble the burgers on rolls with the yogurt sauce, cucumber, tomato and onion.

Servings: 4 / Yield: 4 burgers

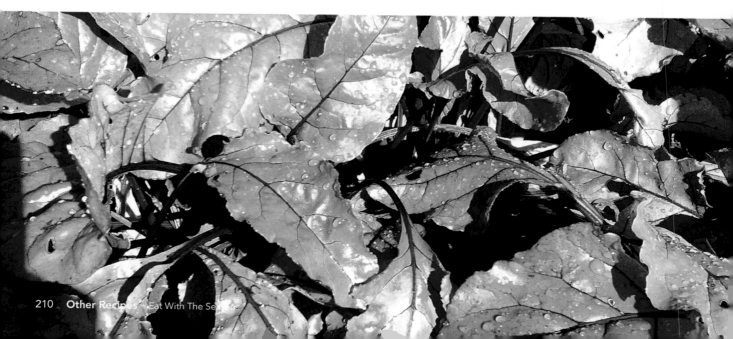

KALE CHIPS

This is the easiest and tastiest snack for times when you are in a hurry. Try any combination of spices, or no spice at all.

- 2 bunches of kale, washed and dried
- ½ teaspoon paprika
- ¼ teaspoon salt
- Dash of cayenne pepper
- 2 tablespoons olive oil

▶ Preheat the oven to 350°F.

▶ Wash and dry kale. Remove leaves from stems and rip into chip-sized pieces. Place kale in large bowl.

▶ Drizzle about 2 tablespoons of olive oil on kale and evenly massage onto leaves. Slowly add salt and paprika and pepper (or your choice of seasonings) to kale while tossing in bowl. (You can also put the kale in a plastic bag with other ingredients and mix together.)

▶ Spread kale evenly on very lightly coated baking sheet or on parchment paper on baking sheet. Place in the oven and bake for about 12 minutes. Flip after 5 minutes. Keep your eye on them to make sure they don't over cook or burn (which can happen quickly).

▶ Remove when done and place on paper towels to absorb excess oil. It will be hard not to eat them all at once. They don't store very well because they tend to get wilted.

Servings: 6

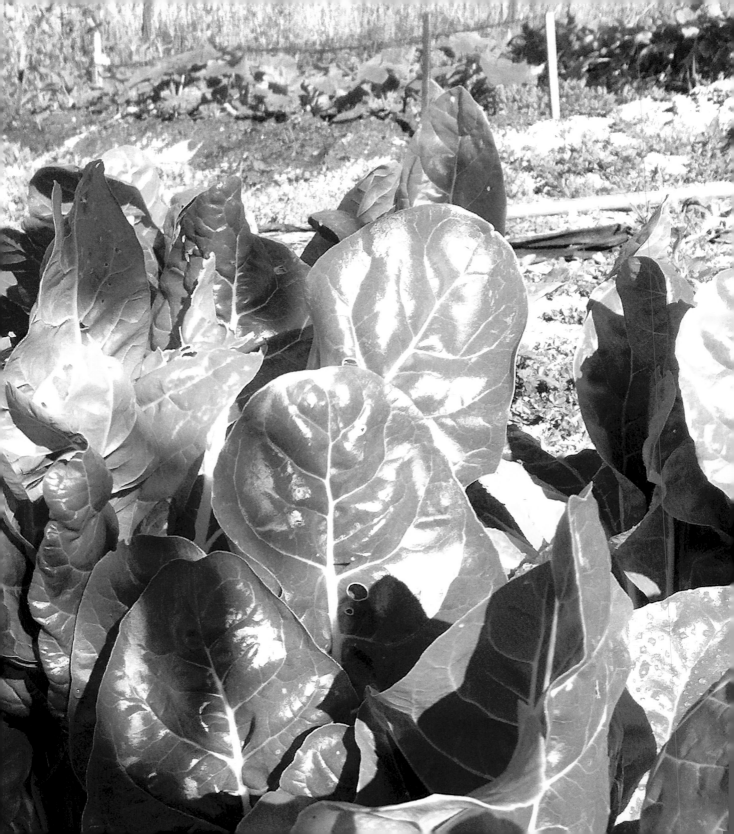

Orange Millet Pilaf

This is a great pilaf for anyone but also those who are gluten intolerant. It comes from Annemarie Colbin's repertoire of whole food recipes. It's easy to make and pairs well with vegetables or stew.

- 3 oranges, plus their juice
- 2 to 3 cups water or vegetable stock
- 2½ cups millet
- ½ teaspoon sea salt
- 2 tablespoons unrefined sesame oil, or unsalted butter
- Freshly ground nutmeg to taste (or substitute ground nutmeg)
- ½ cup walnuts, (optional)

▶ Grate the rind of the oranges and set aside. Juice the oranges, measure , and add enough water or stock to make 4 cups plus 2 tablespoons liquid; set aside.

▶ Wash and drain the millet. In a 3- to 4-quart heavy stainless-steel pot, dry-roast the millet over high heat, stirring continuously, for about 10 minutes, or until fragrant.

▶ Add the liquid to the saucepan along with the salt. Bring to a boil, reduce heat, and simmer for 30 minutes, covered.

▶ While the millet is cooking, heat the butter or oil, in a small skillet, add the grated orange rind, nutmeg, and walnuts. Stir once and remove from heat.

▶ Fold into the cooked millet. Serve immediately.

Servings: 8

Poached Halibut or Salmon

I learned this recipe from Chef Peter Berley and it is so delicious and easy to do.

- 2 quarts water
- 1 cup dry white wine
- 1 lemon, thinly sliced
- 1 sprig parsley
- 1 teaspoon black peppercorns
- 2 tablespoons sea salt
- 1½ pound halibut fillet (salmon)

▶ Combine the water, wine and remaining ingredients (except fish) in a wide enough pan to hold the fish. Bring to a boil then lower the heat and simmer 10 minutes. Add the fish and cook at a gentle simmer. Do not allow the liquid to boil. Cover and poach for 5 to 7 minutes until barely cooked through. Turn off the heat and allow the fish to finish cooking for several minutes. Transfer the fish to a platter. Blot the excess moisture from the fish.

Servings: 4

Raw Kale Salad

I ate a salad similar to this at a restaurant in New York City and it was so delicious that I had to make a version for myself.

- 1 bunch raw kale, chopped
- 2 tablespoons extra virgin olive oil
- 1 tablespoon freshly squeezed lime juice
- ½ teaspoon ginger, grated

- ½ cup dried cranberries
- 2 tablespoons red onion, chopped
- ¼ cup toasted walnuts, or pine nuts
- Sea salt and ground pepper

▶ Mix the chopped kale with the olive oil, lime juice and ginger until well coated.

▶ Add the cranberries and onions, salt and pepper, and toss. Top with walnuts and serve.

Refried Beans

This is an easy recipe for using leftover beans so I like to cook extra just to make this.

- 3 cups dried pinto beans, soaked
- 6 cups water
- 1 bay leaf
- 1 carrot
- 1 teaspoon sea salt
- 3 medium onions

- 3 tablespoons extra virgin olive oil
- 1 heaping teaspoon dried oregano
- 1 heaping teaspoon dried basil
- 1 tablespoon cumin
- Your favorite hot sauce (optional)

▶ Drain the beans. Place them in a 4-quart pot. Add the 6 cups water or enough to cover by 1-inch. Add the bay leaf and carrot.Bring to a boil, reduce heat, and simmer, covered, for 45 minutes, or until the beans are soft. Add the salt and cook for 10 minutes more, then remove the carrot and bay leaf. Drain the beans, reserving the cooking liquid.

▶ Chop the onions and you should have about 2 cups. In a large skillet, heat the oil, add the onions and sauté over medium heat for about 6 to 8 minutes, or until soft. Add the oregano, basil, and cumin.

▶ Continue to sauté for 5 minutes more, adding about ¼ cup of the bean liquid so that the onions do not burn. When the onions are sweet and soft, add the beans and mash to a thick paste. Cook over low heat, uncovered for about 5 to 8 minutes, adding bean liquid as necessary to keep the beans from drying out and burning. If you wish, season with Tabasco or hot sauce to taste. Serve hot.

Servings: 8

SHRIMP IN PARCHMENT

This is a similar version to the chicken / fish in parchment with just a few changes to the spices. Just as easy to make though. I love using coconut oil with shrimp. It adds a nice flavor.

- 1½ tablespoon tamari or shoyu
- 2 limes, juiced
- 1 tablespoon hoisin sauce (or other hot sauce) **OR** 2 mild chili peppers, seeded and sliced
- 1 teaspoon sesame oil (can be spicy if preferred)
- 1½ tablespoon rice vinegar
- 1 teaspoon honey
- 3 cloves garlic, minced
- 1, 1-inch strip fresh ginger (or to taste), minced

- 3 tablespoons sesame, coconut, or olive oil
- 1½ pound jumbo shrimp, peeled and deveined
- 4 heads baby bok choy, rinsed and trimmed (or 2 large)
- 1 bunch asparagus spears, trimmed
- 2 tablespoons scallions, thinly sliced
- ¼ cup cilantro, chopped
- Sea salt and pepper to taste

▶ Preheat oven to 375°F. Position racks in upper and lower thirds of the oven. Prepare 4 parchment sheets.

▶ In a bowl mix the first six ingredients, through honey, until blended.

▶ In a medium bowl, combine the shrimp, ginger, and garlic. Pour about half of the tamari mixture over the shrimp and toss to coat.

▶ In another medium bowl, combine the bok choy, scallions, any other vegetables you are using, and cilantro. Add the remaining tamari mixture to the bowl and toss to coat.

▶ Fold the parchment paper in half and open up. Brush the inside with oil if desired. Place baby bok choy on the bottom (on the crease), pouring remaining liquid over top. Then place shrimp on top and any other vegetables that you might be adding to your parchment, like the broccoli or asparagus. Top with the liquid mixture and salt and pepper to taste. Fold up the parchment and seal with a paperclip.

▶ Place parchment packs on a baking sheet and in the oven for about 8 minutes. Switch positions of the baking sheets and bake for another 7 minutes, or until the packets are puffed. Remove packets from the oven — open carefully to let the steam escape — and transfer to serving plates. Serve with rice, couscous, or quinoa.

Servings: 6

SNAPPY SALMON BURGERS

Another easy recipe that you can make from canned salmon for a quick meal, or use fresh leftover salmon. Since salmon is so loaded with essential fatty acids, vitamin E and protein, I had to include some easy salmon recipes for dinner. Remember to always use wild caught Pacific salmon for sustainability and health reasons.

- ⅓ cup green onion chopped
- ¼ cup cilantro, chopped
- ½ jalapeño pepper, seeded and diced
- ½ lime, freshly squeezed
- ¼ teaspoon sea salt
- ½ cup breadcrumbs, (natural brand without additives like Panko*)
- 1 teaspoon Dijon style mustard
- 1 can (14-ounce) wild Alaskan salmon packed in water, without bones or skin, drained

▶ Place onions, cilantro, chili pepper, and lime juice in a food processor; process until finely chopped. Add salt and salmon; pulse 4 times or until salmon is coarsely ground and mixture is well blended.

▶ Divide salmon mixture into 4 equal portions; shape each portion into a 1-inch thick burger. If not cooking right away cover and chill in refrigerator.

▶ Heat olive oil in a pan over medium heat. Add the burgers and cook for about 6 minutes on each side and they are browned.

▶ Serve burgers with the herbed yogurt spread or mango ketchup.

* For a Gluten-free option, substitute almond meal.

Servings: 4

Socca Pancake (Chickpea Pancake)

This is such an easy and delicious treat. My first taste of socca was when I was very young and we lived in France in the Nice area. They make it in little pizza type shops in the old part of the city in the giant wood ovens, wrap it in paper, salt it, and serve it nice and warm. A French version of fast food! I love it because it's made from chickpea flour, so gluten free! I found this recipe in my favorite cookbook by Martha Rose Shulman, Mediterranean Light. SO YUMMY!!!!

- ⅔ cup chickpea flour
- ¼ to ½ teaspoon sea salt
- 1 cup cold water
- 2 tablespoons olive oil
- Freshly ground pepper

▶ Thirty minutes before baking, preheat the oven to 475°F. Brush a pizza pan or heavy baking dish or cast iron enameled skillet with 1 tablespoon of olive oil.

▶ Beat together the flour, salt and water until there are no lumps, (which can also be done in the blender at high speed). Add freshly ground pepper to taste. Let sit for 30 minutes.

▶ Heat the oiled baking pan in the pre heated oven for about 10 to 15 minutes, until it's good and hot, then pour in the batter. It should be about ¼-inch thick. Drizzle the remaining oil over the top of the batter. Set in the upper third of the oven and bake for about 5 minutes, until set. Place the pan under the broiler and brown for 3 to 4 minutes, turning the pan several times. Remove from the heat and scrape out servings with a spatula. It may stick a little.

Tip: This can also be used as a roll up for vegetables or hummus. It makes a great lunch or snack.

Servings: 6

SOCCA (CHICKPEA PANCAKE) CRÊPES

This is a similar recipe to the socca snack but for use as a crêpe. They have a nutty flavor and are great for gluten-free dinners. Try stuffing with roasted vegetables and topping with a garlic basil oil.

- 2 large eggs
- ⅔ cup milk (rice or regular)
- 2 tablespoons extra virgin olive oil
- ½ cup chickpea flour
- 2 tablespoons corn flour (masa harina)
- ½ teaspoon sea salt

▶ Blend together the eggs, milk and oil. Slowly add the flour and salt mixing with wooden spoon. Blend for 1 minute. Set aside in a bowl or large glass measuring cup for 30 minutes or longer.

For individual crêpes:

▶ Heat a well-seasoned crepe pan over medium heat and brush lightly with olive oil. Ladle in about 2 tablespoons of batter per crepe. It should sizzle when it hits the pan so quickly tilt the pan to distribute the batter evenly. Cook on the first side for about 1 minute. Turn the crepe and brown on the other side for about 30 seconds. Transfer to a plate and continue with the remaining batter, stacking the crepes as they are done. Eat plain, with salt, or stuff with your favorite vegetables. To reheat, wrap in foil and heat in 350°F oven.

For a giant crêpe:

▶ Heat a well-seasoned cast iron skillet over medium high heat and brush with olive oil. Ladle in the batter and tilt the pan to distribute evenly. Cook on the first side until it begins to brown. Turn the crepe by sliding it onto a dish and flipping it over and into the pan again. You can also cook it in the oven at 375°F until brown and crispy on the top. Serve immediately with salt and pepper.

Servings: 6

White Bean Salad with Sun-Dried Tomatoes

This is a nice warm salad that gets a lot of its flavor from the smoked mozzarella. I often use smoked Gouda as well.

- ½ cup extra virgin olive oil
- 1 cup red onion, diced
- ½ teaspoon coarse sea salt or kosher salt
- 1 cup carrots (about 2 medium), peeled and thinly sliced
- 1 cup celery chopped
- 2 cloves garlic, minced
- 2 tablespoons fresh rosemary, minced
- ½ teaspoon crushed red pepper
- 1 can (15-ounce) white beans, rinsed and drained
- ½ cup sun-dried tomatoes, oil packed
- ¼ pound smoked mozzarella, diced
- ¼ cup red wine vinegar (or ume plum vinegar)
- 2 tablespoons flat-leafed parsley, finely chopped, for garnish
- 4 cups arugula leaves, for serving

▶ In a large sauté pan over high heat, combine the oil, onion, and ½ teaspoon of salt and sauté for 2 minutes. Add the carrots, celery, garlic, rosemary, and red pepper flakes and sauté for 1 more minute. Add ¼ cup of water and cover the pan. Cook over high heat until the vegetables are just crisp-tender, about 2 minutes.

▶ Uncover the pan and turn off the heat. Stir in the beans, tomatoes, mozzarella, and vinegar, and season with salt.

▶ Serve on a bed of arugula and garnished with chopped parsley.

    Servings: 8

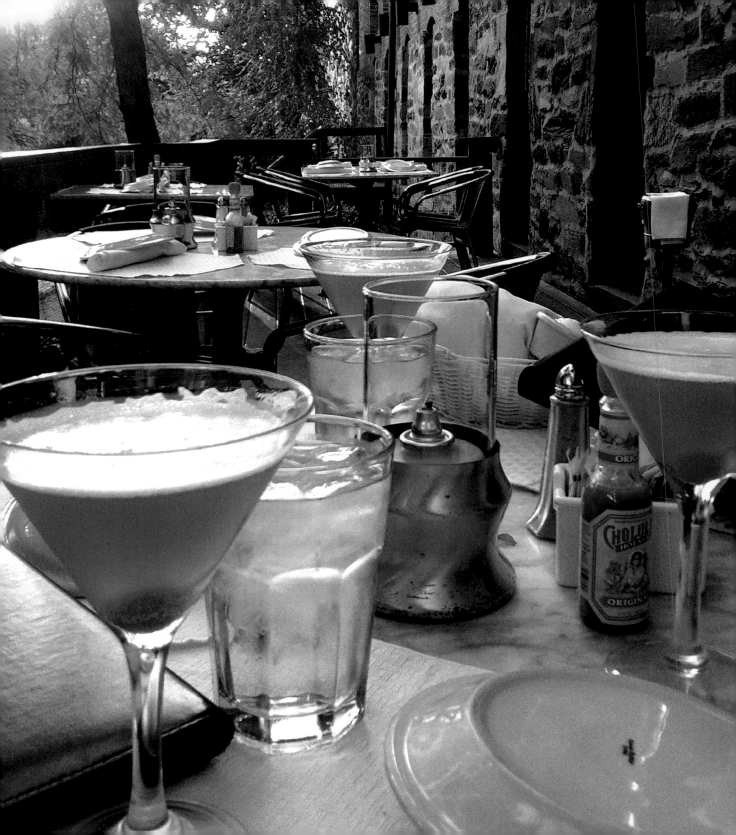

BEVERAGES

ALMOND MILK

This is an easy version for your own almond milk. You can make it in batches and freeze.
I like to use this for my smoothies.

- 5 almonds soaked overnight in about 1 cup of water
- 2 cups water
- ½ teaspoon ground cardamom or vanilla (optional)

▶ In the morning, drain the almonds, place in a blender with water and blend until pulverized. Strain through a fine sieve. Add vanilla or cardamom if desired. Use immediately or freeze for future use.

Servings: 1

B-VITAMIN BOOST

Great boost for the vegetarian diet.

- ½ cup orange juice
- 1 cup chopped pineapple
- ¼ cup rice milk
- ¼ cup apricots, peaches or nectarines, pitted and chopped
- 1 banana, peeled and sliced
- 2 tablespoons wheat germ
- 2 teaspoons ground flaxseed
- 1 teaspoon cod liver oil, flaxseed oil or hemp oil

▶ In a blender, combine orange juice, pineapple, milk, apricots, banana, wheat germ, flaxseed and oil. Cover with lid and blend on low for 30 seconds. Gradually increase speed to high and blend for 30 seconds or until smooth.

Servings: 4

KOMBU & GINGER TEA

This is a wonderfully warming digestive tea to calm and nourish your system.

- 1 tablespoon kombu, in pieces
- 2 cups water
- ¼ teaspoon fresh ginger, grated
- 1 teaspoon honey, optional
- ¼ teaspoon green tea leaves, optional

▶ Bring water to just boiling.

▶ Pour over kombu and ginger and steep for 2 minutes. Add green tea leaves and steep for 3 more minutes.

▶ Strain and serve warm. Add honey if desired.

Servings: 1 / Yield: 1 cup

LAVENDER LEMONADE

I learned how to make this recipe at the Lavender Festival in, of all places, York, Pennsylvania. It's very refreshing and adds a nice twist to sweet lemonade.

- 1 container frozen, organic lemonade
- 1 quart lavender water
- Ice

▶ To make the lavender water, bring 1 quart of water to a boil, add in ½ cup lavender flowers. Let it boil for 5 minutes, turn off the heat and let it steep for about 15 minutes. Let cool.

▶ Pour contents of the lemonade into your pitcher. Add two containers of cold water and the quart of the lavender water. Stir and serve over ice.

Yield: 2 quarts

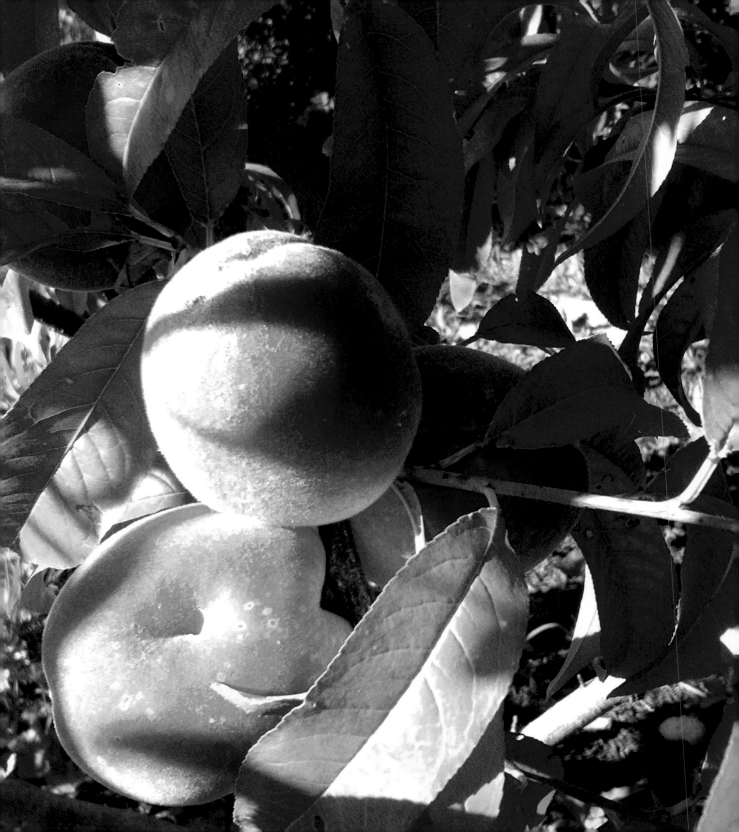

DESSERTS

*"You don't have to cook fancy or complicated masterpieces
— just good food from fresh ingredients."*

— JULIA CHILD

NATURAL SWEETENERS

I must admit that I have always savored my sweets. I enjoyed the search to find alternative ways of eating them because I did not want to give sweet treats up entirely. My biggest weakness has been ice cream but I also love dark chocolate. I believe our culture has a problem with chronic disease mainly because sugar has moved from the "treat" category and into the "staple" file. Not good!! The issue with table sugar (as we know it), is that all the nutrients have been processed out of it. This causes a problem when we eat it because the sugar robs the body of essential nutrients in order to metabolize. There are other natural sweeteners that actually contain trace minerals and nutrients which prevents this process from occurring. So, if you're going to eat sweet, why not work with these natural choices. But remember, sugar is sugar, and too much of it will harm your health whether it's natural or not. Keep it in your diet as a "treat" to savor and you should be fine. I have studied and worked with the natural sweeteners I mention here. I will give you a description and you can decide for yourself which ones you prefer.

BLACKSTRAP MOLASSES: This contains significant amounts of vitamins and minerals. "First" molasses is left over when sugarcane juice is boiled, cooled and removed of its crystals. Blackstrap comes from the third boiling of the sugar syrup and is the most nutritious molasses, containing substantial amounts of calcium, magnesium, potassium, and iron. It has a very strong flavor so it is best to just replace a small portion of sugar with molasses. Consider buying organic because of pesticide concentrations.

RAPADURA: This is Portuguese for unrefined dried sugar cane juice. The least refined of all sugarcane products, it is made simply by cooking juice that has been pressed from sugarcane until it is very concentrated and then drying and granulating it. The only thing that has been removed from the sugarcane is water so it contains all the vitamins and minerals that are normally in the sugarcane juice, namely iron. It replaces sugar 1:1 and adds a dark color and a bit of molasses flavor so it's best for baked goods.

SUCANAT: Stands for SUgar-CAne-NATural and is very similar to Rapadura. It is made by mechanically extracting sugarcane juice, which is then heated and cooled until tiny brown crystals form. Replaces sugar 1:1 and can be an accepted substitute for brown sugar.

TURBINADO SUGAR: After the sugarcane is pressed to extract the juice, the juice is then boiled, cooled, and allowed to crystallize into granules (like Sucanat). But next, these granules are refined to a light tan color by washing them in a centrifuge to remove impurities and surface molasses. It is lighter in color and contains less molasses than Rapadura and Sucanat. A popular brand is Sugar in the Raw. Replaces sugar 1:1 and also a good substitute for brown sugar.

EVAPORATED CANE JUICE: This is basically a finer, lighter-colored version of turbinado sugar. Less refined than table sugar, it also contains trace minerals, including Vitamin B12. Replaces sugar 1:1. Can be used in a wide variety of foods without affecting the color.

STEVIA: This is the most natural sweetener of all. Stevia comes from a South American herb, *Stevia Rebaudiana*, and has been used as a natural sweetener for centuries. The leaves of the plant have a very sweet taste, 25- to 30 times sweeter than sugar, zero glycemic index, zero calories and zero carbs. It is far more healthy than other sweeteners because you eat the whole leaf in powder form. I have grown it in my garden with very good luck, although it is an annual in our area. Because it is so sweet the substitutions vary and, rather than using cups, you use teaspoons and tablespoons. I highly recommend purchasing a cookbook that uses stevia as the sweetener in order to get correct measurements.

BROWN RICE SYRUP: This is made when cooked rice is cultured with enzymes, which break down the starch in the rice. The resulting liquid is cooked down to a thick syrup, which is about half as sweet as white sugar and has a mild butterscotch flavor. It is composed of about 50 percent complex carbohydrates, which break down more slowly in the bloodstream then simple carbs resulting in a less dramatic spike in blood glucose levels. To replace one cup of sugar, use 1⅓ cups brown rice syrup, and for each cup added, reduce liquid by ¼ cups and add ¼ teaspoon baking soda. It has a tendency to make food crispier.

MAPLE SYRUP: Comes from the sap of maple trees, which is collected, filtered, and boiled down to an extremely sweet syrup. It contains fewer calories and a higher concentration of minerals than honey. Don't be fooled by fake maple syrups like Aunt Jemima or Buttersworth. Just read the ingredients because there is nothing but maple syrup in the real thing. To replace 1 cup of sugar use about ¾ cups syrup and lower the oven temperature by 25°F. For each cup of syrup reduce liquid by about 2 tablespoons.

HONEY: Made by the bees from the nectar of flowers, it is ready-made and contains traces of nutrients. To replace 1 cup of sugar use about ⅔ cups honey and lower the oven by 25°F. Reduce liquids by about 2 tablespoons for each cup of honey. I prefer not to cook with honey as it destroys the B Vitamins.

APPLE CRISP

Apple Crisp is one of my all time favorite fruit desserts because it's juicy and light. Sometimes I even eat it for breakfast! I love changing up the fruit according to the season and using rhubarb and strawberries, pears, or plums. It's quick and easy and makes the kitchen smell wonderful.

- 1 cup rolled oats
- ½ cup whole wheat pastry flour
- ½ teaspoon sea salt
- ¼ cup coconut oil (or 5 tablespoons melted butter)
- ¼ cup real maple syrup
- 1½ cups chopped nuts (almonds, walnuts, pecans. brazil nuts)
- ½ cup sunflower seeds and sesame seeds

- 2 tablespoons real maple syrup
- 1 teaspoon cinnamon
- ¼ teaspoon nutmeg
- 2 teaspoons vanilla
- 6 cups apples, cored and sliced into 8 wedges each
- 2 teaspoons arrowroot, for thickening (optional)

▶ Preheat oven to 350°F.

▶ Mix oats, flour, salt in a bowl.

▶ Add oil (or butter) and ¼ cup of maple syrup. Mix well.

▶ Stir in nuts and seeds and set aside.

▶ In a small bowl combine the 2 tablespoons of syrup, spices, and vanilla, set aside.

▶ Prepare fruit and place in a lightly oiled or buttered baking dish. Sprinkle with arrowroot (if using). Pour the liquid mixture over the fruit and toss gently.

▶ Spoon the oat nut mixture over the fruit, cover and bake 45 minutes. Uncover and bake 15 minutes more to crisp.

Servings: 12

APPLE UPSIDE-DOWN CAKE

I love this recipe for special occasions. It is so sweet and moist with a delicious nutty flavor. The honey flavor is important so I like to try different types of local honeys for variation. My favorite was the lavender honey I purchased in France one year.

- 3 apples, peeled, cored and sliced about ¼-inch thick
- 4 tablespoons lavender or other flavorful honey
- ¼-pound (½ cup) plus 3 tablespoons unsalted butter at room temperature
- ¾ cup honey
- 1 teaspoon vanilla

- ¼ teaspoon almond extract
- 3 eggs at room temperature
- ⅔ cups blanched almonds, finely ground
- 1 cup unbleached, unbromated flour
- 1 teaspoon baking powder
- ¼ teaspoon sea salt and/or Kosher salt

▶ Preheat oven to 375°F. Prepare apples ahead. Heat 3 tablespoons butter in a 10-inch cast iron skillet over medium heat. Add the 4 tablespoons of honey and bring to a slight boil, and let cook gently over medium heat until the honey turns a shade darker and begins to caramelize. Immediately arrange apples on the caramel, overlapping them on the outer edge of the pan, then reversing direction, filling in the center.

▶ For the cake, cream the butter until light and fluffy, add the ¾ cups of honey and mix well, then add vanilla and almond extract. Beat in the eggs one at a time until smooth. Stir in the nut flour, followed by the remaining ingredients. Spoon the batter over the apples and smooth it out with a spatula.

▶ Bake in the center of the oven until the cake is golden and springy when pressed with a fingertip, about 35 minutes. Let cool in the pan for a few minutes, then set a cake plate on top of the pan, grasp both the plate and the pan tightly, and turn it over. Carefully ease the pan off the cake. If any fruit sticks to the pan, just take it off and place it on the cake.

Servings: 10

CHEWY BANANA OAT COOKIES

- 1½ cups oats
- ½ cup oat flour or millet flour
- ½ teaspoon salt
- ¼ teaspoon baking soda
- Dash of ground cinnamon (optional)
- ½ cup of chopped nuts and/or raisins
- 2 medium bananas, mashed (about 1 cup)
- ⅓ cup coconut oil, melted or at room temperature
- ½ cup dark chocolate chips

▶ Preheat oven to 350°F. Mix dry ingredients.

▶ In a separate bowl, mix mashed bananas and oil, then add to the dry ingredients. Stir in nuts/raisins and chocolate chips. Drop by the heaping teaspoons on a non-oiled cookie sheet. Bake 10 to 15 minutes. Makes about 2 dozen cookies.

Servings: 12

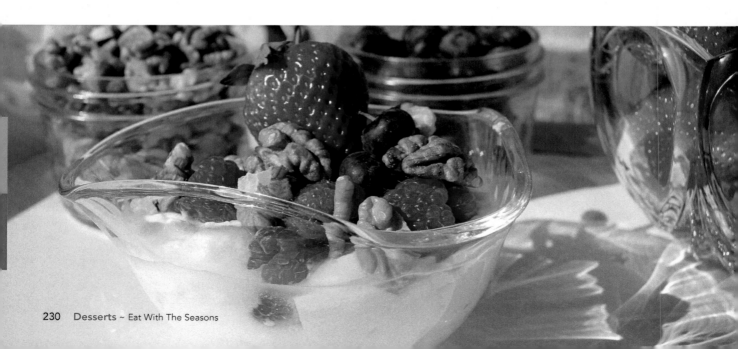

CHOCOLATE WALNUT COOKIES

This is a nice cookie with a chocolate flavor that will satisfy a sweet tooth and a chocolate craving.

- 1 cup spelt flour
- ½ cup natural cocoa
- ½ teaspoon baking soda
- ¼ teaspoon baking powder
- ¼ teaspoon salt
- 6 tablespoon unsalted butter, at room temperature (or use coconut oil for a nice flavor)
- 2 tablespoons olive oil
- ½ cup organic sucanat sugar
- 1 large egg
- 1 teaspoon vanilla extract
- ¾ cup walnuts, chopped
- ¾ cups dark chocolate chips (optional)

▶ Preheat oven to 350°F. Line two baking sheets with parchment paper.

▶ In a medium bowl, combine flour, cocoa, baking soda, baking powder, and salt. Mix thoroughly with a wire whisk. Set aside.

▶ In a stand mixer, or in a bowl with a hand mixer, beat the butter and oil on medium speed until creamy. Add sugar, beating until well combined. Beat in the egg and vanilla. Turn the mixer to low speed (or with a wooden spoon), and mix in the flour mixture just until incorporated. Mix in the nuts and chocolate chips if using.

▶ Drop heaping teaspoonfuls of batter about 1½ inches apart on the prepared baking sheets. Bake for 9 to 11 minutes, watching carefully that they don't burn on the bottom. After 5 minutes rotate the pans from front to back so that they cook evenly. The cookies will puff up and then settle down slightly when done. Let cool on the baking sheets on a wire rack for a few minutes. With a metal spatula, transfer the cookies to a rack to cool completely.

Servings: 24

Cocoa Beanie Squares

Great sweet alternative that will balance a sweet tooth. The "secret" ingredient gives this dessert lots of protein and fiber. The kids will love this. Just don't tell them what is in it!

- 1½ to 2 cups dark chocolate chips
- 2 cups Adzuki beans, drained and rinsed
- 4 eggs
- ¾ cup brown rice syrup
- ½ teaspoon baking powder

▶ Melt chocolate chips in double boiler.

▶ In blender or food processor, combine beans and eggs.

▶ Add syrup, baking powder, and chocolate, process until very smooth.

▶ Pour batter into a 9x9-inch or 8x8-inch non-stick or oiled pan.

▶ Bake for 45 minutes. Let cool and serve.

Servings: 16

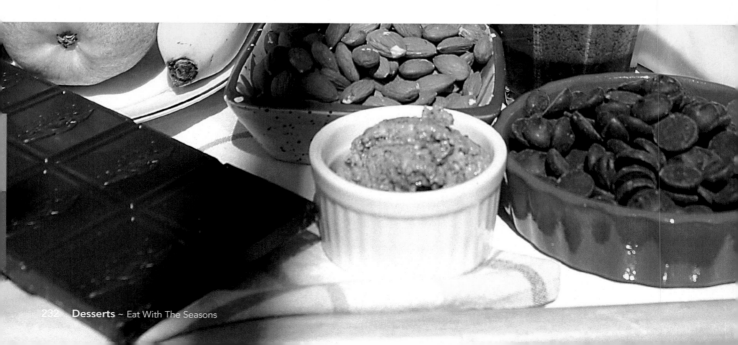

MOLASSES GINGER COOKIES

These are my favorite cookies. I love the molasses paired with the crystallized ginger pieces. They can be baked a little longer for a crisper cookie that is more like a ginger snap but I like them a little under-cooked for a chewier texture.

- ¼ cup unsalted butter, softened
- 1 cup, plus ⅓ cup organic sugar like turbinado, sucanat or rapadura, divided
- 1 large egg, beaten
- ¼ cup molasses
- 2 cups spelt flour
- 2 teaspoons baking soda
- 1 teaspoon ground cinnamon
- ½ teaspoon salt
- ¼ teaspoon ground cloves
- ⅛ teaspoon ground ginger
- ⅓ cup crystallized ginger, finely chopped

▶ In a large bowl, beat the butter and 1 cup of the sucanat sugar with an electric mixer until creamy. Add the egg and molasses. Mix well.

▶ In another bowl, whisk flour, baking soda, cinnamon, salt, cloves, and ginger until well blended. Add the dry ingredients to the wet ingredients. Stir in the crystallized ginger. Mix well, until it is all incorporated. Chill the dough in the refrigerator until firm, 30 minutes to 1 hour.

▶ Preheat oven to 375°F. Cover 2 baking sheets with parchment paper.

▶ Roll the dough into 1-inch balls and then roll in the sugar. Place 1½ inches apart on the prepared baking sheet.

▶ Bake the cookies, in batches, until they crackle on top, 8 to 10 minutes.

▶ Transfer to a wire rack to cool.

Servings: 12 / Yield: 3 dozen

Oatmeal Chocolate Chip Walnut Cookies

This is my substitute for the original chocolate chip cookies. These are quick to make without all the sugar. Great for kids and to serve to guests, but are still a healthier version for you to enjoy in small portions.

- 1½ cups rolled oats
- 1 cup spelt flour (or whole wheat pastry flour)
- ¼ teaspoon sea salt
- ¼ teaspoon baking powder
- ⅔ cup real maple syrup

- ½ cup melted butter (or coconut oil)
- 1 teaspoon vanilla
- 1 egg
- ½ cup chopped walnuts (optional) or almonds
- ½ cup good quality dark chocolate chips

▶ Preheat oven to 350°F. Combine oats, flour, salt, and baking powder together in a bowl; set aside.

▶ In a separate bowl, mix together sweetener, butter or oil, vanilla, egg and maple syrup. Add wet ingredients to dry mixture and mix well.

▶ Stir in nuts and chips.

▶ With moist hands form dough into 3-inch cookies and place on a lightly oiled cookie sheet or one lined with parchment paper.

▶ Bake for 8 to 10 minutes, until golden brown.

Servings: 24

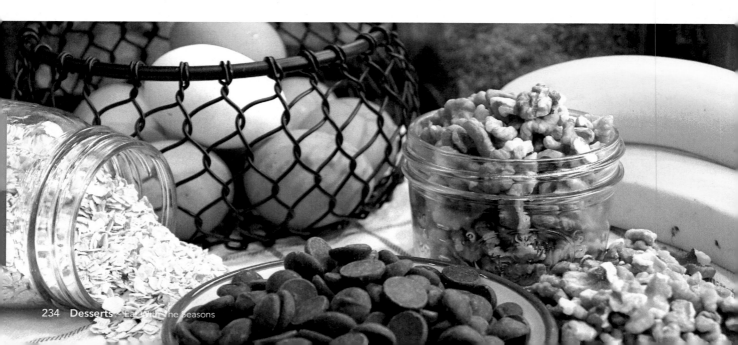

OATMEAL, PECAN, CRANBERRY COOKIES

This is a nice cookie to make in the fall when cranberries and oatmeal feel right. They are not overly sweet and the chocolate adds just the right amount of sweetness.

- 1¼ cups spelt flour
- 1 cup rolled oats
- ¾ teaspoon baking powder
- ½ teaspoon baking soda
- ½ teaspoon salt
- ½ cup organic turbinado sugar
- ½ cup pure maple syrup
- ⅓ cup organic butter, softened
  (or substitute coconut oil for a nice flavor)
- 1½ teaspoon vanilla extract
- 1 large egg
- ½ cup applesauce
- ¾ cup chopped pecans, toasted
- ½ cup dark chocolate chips
- 1 cup dried cranberries

▶ Preheat oven to 350°F.

▶ Combine flour and next 4 ingredients (through salt), stirring with a whisk. Set aside.

▶ Place sugars and butter in a large bowl; beat with a mixer at medium speed until well blended. Add vanilla and egg; beat until blended. Add applesauce and stir. Gradually add flour mixture, beating at low speed just until combined. Stir in pecans, cranberries and chocolate chips.

▶ Drop by tablespoonfuls 2 inches apart onto baking sheets lined with parchment paper. Bake at 350°F for 12 minutes or until edges of cookies are lightly browned. Cool on the pans 2 minutes. Remove cookies from pans; cool on wire racks.

Servings: 36

STRAWBERRY-RHUBARB CRISP

I love swapping out the fruit depending on the season, and using the same topping.

- 1 cup rolled oats
- ½ cup spelt flour
- 1½ cups almond or walnut flour
- ½ teaspoon cinnamon
- ¼ teaspoon salt
- ½ cup sunflower seeds
- ⅓ cup maple syrup
- 1 teaspoon vanilla extract

- ¼ cup coconut oil
  (or 5 tablespoons melted butter)
- ¼ teaspoon salt
- 3 cups rhubarb, heated
- ½ cup turbinado sugar
- 3 cups strawberries, sliced
- ½ teaspoon orange zest, optional

▶ Preheat oven to 350°F.

▶ Stir together oats, flour, nuts, sunflower seeds and cinnamon in a medium bowl.

▶ Whisk together the maple syrup, vanilla extract, coconut oil (or butter) and salt in another bowl.

▶ Stir the wet into the dry, mixing until liquid is absorbed.

▶ Heat Rhubarb with ½ cup of sugar until cooked, about 8 minutes or so.

▶ Combine cooked rhubarb, strawberries, and orange zest in a bowl and pour into an oiled baking pan (8x8-inch or 9x13-inch). Top with oat mixture and bake for about 25 minutes, until brown and crisped.

Servings: 8

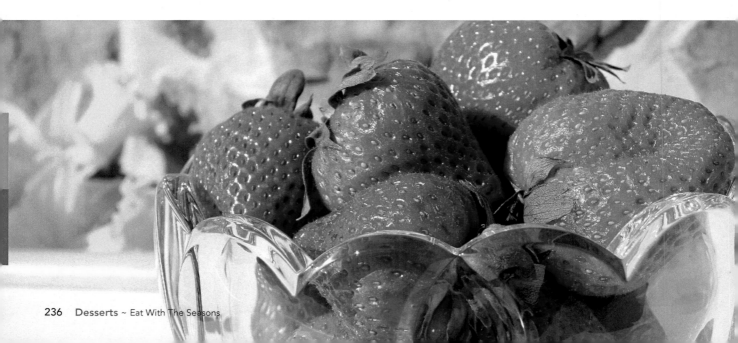

SUMMER PEACH CRISP

There's nothing like juicy summer peaches.

- 1 cup rolled oats
- ½ cup whole wheat pastry flour
- ½ teaspoon sea salt
- 1½ cups chopped nuts (almonds, walnuts, pecans)
- ½ cup sunflower seeds
- ¼ cup real maple syrup
- ¼ cup coconut oil
  (or 5 tablespoons melted butter)
- 2 tablespoon real maple syrup
- 1 teaspoon cinnamon
- ¼ teaspoon nutmeg
- 2 teaspoons vanilla
- 1 pint blueberries
- 3 cups sliced peaches
- 1 to 2 tablespoons arrowroot

▶ Preheat oven to 350°F.

▶ Mix oats, flour, salt in a bowl.

▶ Add oil (or butter) and ¼ cup maple syrup. Mix well.

▶ Stir in nuts and seeds and set aside.

▶ In a small bowl combine the 2 tablespoons of maple syrup, spices, and vanilla, set aside.

▶ Prepare fruit and place in a lightly oiled or buttered baking dish. Sprinkle with arrowroot. Pour the liquid mixture over the fruit and toss gently.

▶ Spoon the oat nut mixture over the fruit, cover and bake 45 minutes. Uncover and bake 15 minutes more to crisp.

Servings: 12

Zucchini Cookies

These are such a delicious little treat for a 4 o'clock pick me up.

- ½ cup butter, softened
- ½ cup honey
- ¼ cup real maple syrup
- 1 egg
- ½ teaspoon vanilla
- 1½ cups spelt flour
- 2 tablespoons wheat germ
- ½ teaspoon baking soda
- ½ teaspoon salt

- 1 cup rolled oats
- 1 teaspoon cinnamon
- 1½ cups shredded zucchini
- 1½ cup granola (homemade or a low-sugar option)
- 1 cup nuts, chopped
- 1 cup dark chocolate chips
- 1 cup dried cranberries

▶ Heat oven to 350°F.

▶ Beat butter and sweeteners in a bowl until fluffy. Add egg and vanilla and mix well.

▶ In a separate bowl, combine flour, wheat germ, baking soda, salt, cinnamon and oats and mix well. Add to sugar mixture and stir well.

▶ Add zucchini, and granola and mix.

▶ Stir in nuts, chocolate chips and cranberries.

▶ Drop by spoonfuls onto a cookie sheet and bake for 10 to 12 minutes until brown on bottom.

Servings: 24 / Yield: 24

Gluten-Free
Dessert Options

Apricot Chewies

These are a nice little snack that I like to bring along when I'm on the go and want something sweet. I like to think of them as "girlie" treats because apricots and molasses provide lots of iron which is often lacking in women, especially teenagers. They also contain Vitamin A which contributes to our body's immune reaction, and calcium which is essential for bone support....all the areas where women seem to require more support. I often add cacao nibs for more magnesium and a little crunch.

- 12 dried apricots, with apple juice for soaking
- 6 dried figs, tough stems removed
- ½ cup raisins
- ½ cup almonds
- ½ cup sunflower seeds
- 2 tablespoons blackstrap molasses
- ½ cup wheat germ**
- Coconut flakes

▶ Soak apricots and figs in apple juice for a few hours or overnight. Drain. (You can retain the juice for another purpose or even drink it).

▶ Combine the apricots, figs, raisins, almonds, seeds, molasses, and wheat germ in a food processor or blender. Process until the ingredients are finely chopped.

▶ Form the batter into a sausage-like roll on wax paper. Cover with coconut flakes. Refrigerate for a few hours, slice and roll into balls. You can also roll in sesame seeds or chopped nuts or cocoa powder.

**Omit for gluten-free option.

Servings: 12 / Yield: 2 dozen

Banana Chocolate Chip Bread- Gluten-Free

- ¼ cuplight tasting olive oil or coconut oil
- 2 large eggs
- 1 teaspoon vanilla
- ⅓ cup milk, (cow, rice, almond)
- ¾ cup bananas (2 medium), mashed
- 2⅓ cups flour blend (see recipe)
- 1½ teaspoon xanthan gum
- 2½ teaspoons baking powder
- 1 teaspoon salt
- 1½ teaspoon cinnamon
- ⅔ cup turbinado sugar
- ¾ cup chocolate chips, good quality
- ½ cup nuts, optional, chopped

▶ Preheat oven to 375°F. Grease three loaf pans.

▶ In a large bowl, thoroughly blend all wet ingredients through milk, with electric mixer. Add in the mashed bananas.

▶ In a smaller bowl, sift together dry ingredients, up to chocolate chips, with a whisk. Add to wet ingredients and blend.

▶ Add in chocolate chips (and nuts, if using) and gently stir. Spoon batter into pans.

▶ Bake 35 to 40 minutes or until top is nicely browned. Remove from oven. Cool pan on wire rack for 10 minutes. Remove bread from pan and finish cooling on wire rack.

Servings: 12 / Yield: 2 slices

Gluten-Free Apple Crisp

- 1 cup rolled oats (gluten-free)
- ½ teaspoon sea salt
- 1½ cups chopped nuts
  (almonds, walnuts, pecans. brazil nuts)
- ½ cup sunflower seeds and sesame seeds
- ¼ cup pure maple syrup
- ¼ cup coconut oil
  (or 5 tablespoons melted butter)

- 2 tablespoons real maple syrup
- 1 teaspoon cinnamon
- ¼ teaspoon nutmeg
- 2 teaspoons vanilla
- 6 cups apples, cored and sliced into
  8 wedges each

▶ Preheat oven to 350°F.

▶ Mix oats and salt in a bowl.

▶ Add oil (or butter) and maple syrup. Mix well.

▶ Stir in nuts and seeds and set aside.

▶ In a small bowl combine the 2 tablespoons of syrup, spices, and vanilla, set aside.

▶ Prepare fruit and place in a lightly oiled or buttered baking dish. Sprinkle with arrowroot.
  Pour the liquid mixture over the fruit and toss gently.

▶ Spoon the oat nut mixture over the fruit, cover and bake 45 minutes. Uncover and bake 15 minutes
  more to crisp.

Servings: 12

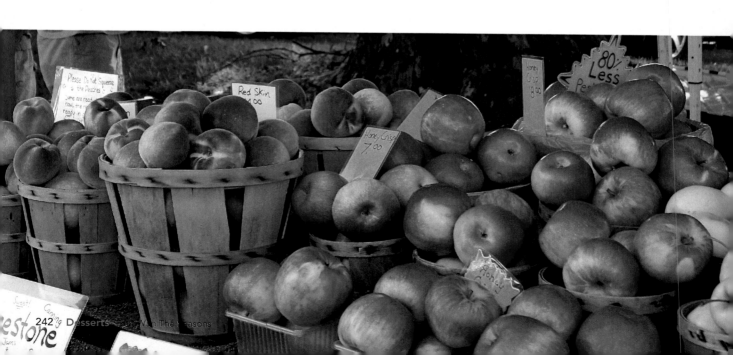

No-Bake Chocolate Chip Cookies

Here's a nice gluten-free and dairy free option that is easy to make. I found this in a magazine, and although it is similar to my Earth Balls, it does not have peanut butter.

- 1¼ cup raisins
- ½ cup dates, pitted and chopped
- 2 cups whole oats
- 4 tablespoons honey

- 1 teaspoon cinnamon
- Pinch sea salt
- ½ cup cacao nibs

▶ Put raisins and dates in the food processor and chop into small pieces. Add oats, honey, cinnamon and salt. Process to mix well.

▶ Empty into a mixing bowl and add cacao nibs. Mix well.

▶ Measure a tablespoon portion and make into a ball and flatten. Or roll in nuts or coconut. Enjoy immediately, or chill for a firmer texture.

Servings: 2 / Yield: 42

Sautéed Apples

What an easy way to eat a warm apple dessert. The combination of apples and cinnamon is a sure sign that fall has arrived. This easy apple recipe gives me all the joy of an apple pie without having to make the dough! I learned this from Chef Peter Berley and decided to substitute maple syrup or honey instead of sugar.

- ¼ cup unsalted butter, at room temperature
- ½ cup honey or maple syrup
- 6 apples, (such as Granny Smith, Gala, Crispin), cored and sliced into wedges

- ¼ cup raisins
- ½ teaspoon cinnamon
- ½ cup apple cider

▶ In a large skillet over high heat, melt the butter. Stir in the honey or maple syrup and cook for 1 minute.

▶ Arrange the apples in a single layer in the pan and scatter the raisins on top. Cook undisturbed for 6 minutes, or until the apples begin to caramelize.

▶ Add the cider and cinnamon, bring to a boil, and cook for 1 minute.

▶ Transfer the apples to a serving dish and serve warm.

Servings: 6

CHOCOLATE EARTH BALLS

These no-cook treats are so rich that it only takes one to satisfy a sweet tooth. Be sure to make them small.

- 1 cup peanut butter, natural, no sugar added
- ⅓ cup honey, mild flavored like clover, or orange blossom
- 2 tablespoons cocoa powder, unsweetened
- ½ cup raisins

- 1 cup coconut, unsweetened, shredded, divided
- ½ cup chocolate chips, good quality, dark
- ¼ cup sesame seeds
- ¼ cup nuts, like almonds or walnuts, finely chopped

▶ Stir up the peanut butter very well before measuring. Mix the peanut butter, honey, and cocoa powder until well combined. Stir in the raisins and only ½ of the coconut. Stir in the chocolate chips. Refrigerate for 1 to 2 hours.

▶ Place the remaining coconut, sesame seeds and nuts into 3 separate bowls. Using a spoon, scoop small spoonfuls of the peanut butter mixture from the bowl, then roll into 1-inch balls. Roll the balls in the coconut or sesame seeds to perfect the shape into a better ball. Roll each finished ball in more of the sesame seeds, chopped nuts, and/or more coconut in whatever combination you prefer.

▶ Arrange the balls on a plate, cover loosely with plastic wrap, and refrigerate for at least 30 minutes before serving.

Servings: 24 / Yield: 24

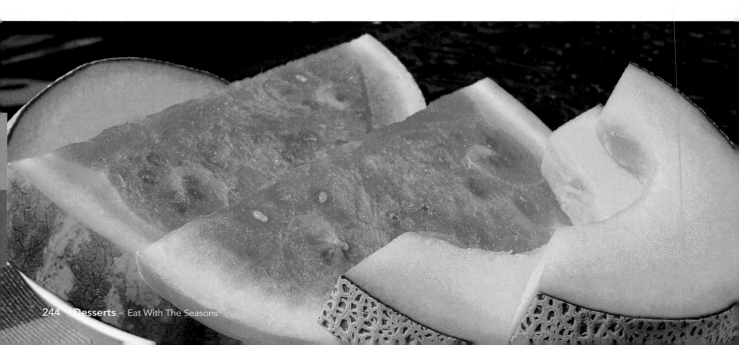

CHERRY NUT CHOCOLATE BARK

This is my favorite chocolate dessert. What a great way to add antioxidants to your diet to help fight free radicals and prevent disease! It makes a great gift for all your chocolate loving friends.

- 12 ounces dark chocolate
- 1 cup almonds, toasted, and chopped. or 1 cup pistachios, toasted, and chopped
- 1 cup unsweetened dried sour cherries
- ¼ cup organic crystallized ginger, chopped
- 1 pinch sea salt

▶ Line a rimmed baking sheet with foil and set aside.

▶ In a double broiler with simmering water, melt the chocolate, stirring frequently, until smooth and melted, about 5 minutes. (You can also melt the chocolate in a bowl set over a saucepan of simmering water.)

▶ Stir in the cherries, ginger, nuts and salt, saving some for decorating the top.

▶ Pour the melted chocolate onto the prepared baking sheet, spreading it with a spatula to about ¼-inch thickness.

▶ Sprinkle evenly with remainder of the chopped ginger, some of the cherries, and nuts for decorative color.

▶ Chill until chocolate is firm, about 30 minutes. Peel off foil and break chocolate into pieces. Store in the refrigerator in an airtight container for up to 1 month. Best served slightly chilled.

Servings: 16

BAKED PEARS

Although these pears have a long cook time, it's worth the wait to have them melt in your mouth. The smell of the cinnamon makes the wait easier to take. This is a nice fall or winter dessert.

- 6 large ripe but firm pears (Bosc pears work well)
- 2 tablespoons honey with a strong flavor like blueberry or orange blossom
- 2 tablespoons turbinado sugar
- 1 teaspoon cinnamon
- 12 cloves
- Water, as needed

▶ Preheat the oven to 400°F. Cut a small cone out of the bottom of each pear and place a teaspoonful of honey in each one. Set the pears, bottom side down, in the baking dish. Sprinkle with water and then sprinkle sugar over tops of each pear. Add the cloves to the baking dish and then add enough water to cover the rounded part of the pears. Add cinnamon to water.

▶ Bake for 10 minutes, then turn down the oven to 350°F. Using a spoon, baste the pears every 15 minutes or so with the juice from the baking dish and bake for 2 hours, or until pears are soft. Turn the pears on their side from time to time so that they cook evenly. Remove from the oven and allow to cool slightly.

▶ Serve the pears at room temperature with some of the leftover syrup drizzled over the top.

Servings: 12

FLOUR BLEND #1

- 1¾ cup rice flour
- 2 cups potato starch
- 1½ cup tapioca starch

RESOURCES & REFERENCES

*Take time to educate yourself and
make informed choices that keep you healthy.*

RESOURCES

- Rodale Institute – www.rodaleinstitute.org
- EWG's Shopper Guide to Pesticides in Produce – www.foodnews.org
- Maine Coast Sea Vegetables – www.seaveg.com

RESOURCES FOR GLUTEN INTOLERANCE

Books
- *Gluten Free 101*, Carol Fenster, Ph.D
- *The Smart Baking Cookbook*, Jane Kinderlehrer
- *Gluten-Free Diet: A Comprehensive Resource Guide*, Shelley Case
- *Wheat Free, Worry Free*, Danna Korn
- *The Gloriously Gluten-Free Cookbook*, Vanessa Maltin

Websites
- www.glutenfreecookingschool.com
- www.celiac.com
- www.enjoylifefoods.com
- www.glutenfree.com

HELPFUL READING
- *The Omnivore's Dilemma*, Michael Pollan – A book about what we should have for dinner and how our choices will determine our survival as a species
- *Nourishing Traditions*, Sally Fallon
- *Animal, Vegetable, Miracle: A Year of Food Life*, Barbara Kingsolver

MOVIES
- Food Inc. – A look inside America's corporate controlled food chain.
- Forks Over Knives – Examines the claim that degenerative diseases that afflict us can be controlled and reversed.
- Food Matters – Documentary about the food we eat that is loaded with chemical additives and nutritionally depleted.

Reference & Notes

- *The Truth about "Natural" Sweeteners: Does Sugar by Any Other Name Still Taste as Sweet?,* Liza Barnes & Nicole Nichols

- *Staying Healthy with the Seasons,* Elson Haas, M.D.

- *Healing with Whole Foods,* Paul Pitchford

- *Food and Healing,* Annemarie Colbin

- *The Natural Gourmet,* Annemarie Colbin

- *Master Your Metabolism,* Jillian Michaels

- *Pediatrics Journal,* March 2008, 121:3, Maureen T. Timlin, Mark A. Pereira, Mary Story, Dianne Neumark-Sztainer

- *Reducing Environmental Cancer Risk, What We Can Do Now,* President's Cancer Panel, LaSAlle Leffall, Jr., M.D.

- *The World's Healthiest Foods,* George Mateljan

- *Seaweed,* Valerie Gennari Cooksley, RN

- *The Seven Steps to Spiritual Success,* Deepak Chopra

- *Fats that Heal, Fats that Kill,* Udo Erasmus

- *The Self Healing Cookbook,* Kristina Turner

- *The Coconut Oil Miracle,* Bruce Fife, CN, ND

- *Old Farmer's Almanac,* www.almanac.com

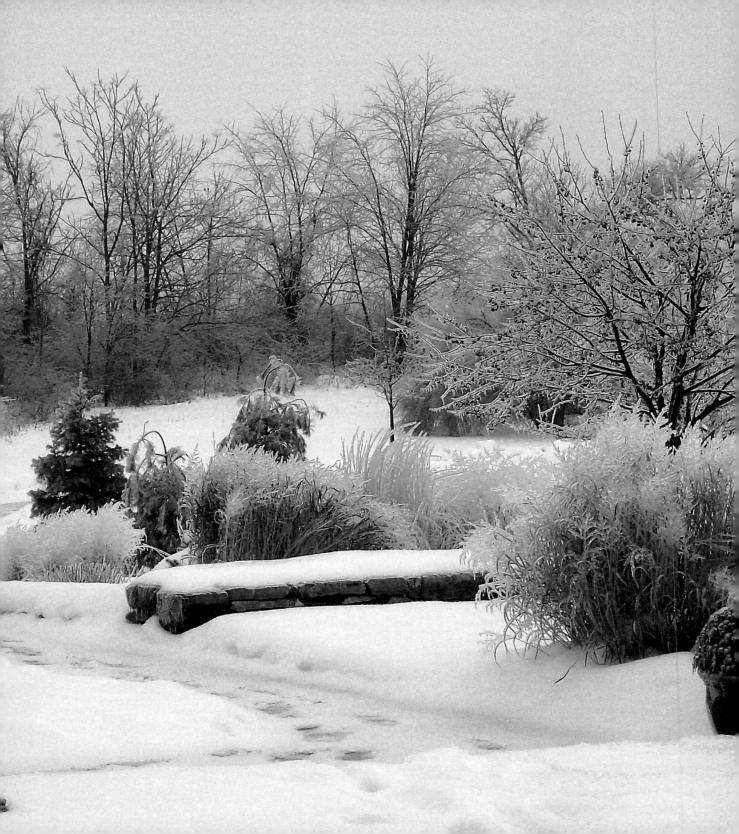

INDEX

INDEX